An Introduction to Forensic Genetics for Non-geneticists

Antonio Amorim

i3S - Institute for Research and Innovation in Health
Porto, Portugal
Biology Department, Faculty of Sciences
University of Porto
Portugal

Nádia Pinto

i3S - Institute for Research and Innovation in Health
Porto, Portugal
CMUP - Center of Mathematics of the University of Porto
Portugal

CRC Press
Taylor & Francis Group
Boca Raton London New York

CRC Press is an imprint of the
Taylor & Francis Group, an **informa** business

A SCIENCE PUBLISHERS BOOK

Cover credit: Image created by the authors of the book.

First edition published 2024
by CRC Press
2385 NW Executive Center Drive, Suite 320, Boca Raton FL 33431

and by CRC Press
4 Park Square, Milton Park, Abingdon, Oxon, OX14 4RN

CRC Press is an imprint of Taylor & Francis Group, LLC

Library of Congress Cataloging-in-Publication Data (applied for)

ISBN: 978-1-032-21096-4 (hbk)
ISBN: 978-1-032-21097-1 (pbk)
ISBN: 978-1-003-26671-6 (ebk)

DOI: 10.1201/9781003266716

Typeset in Palatino Linotype
by Radiant Productions

Foreword – Guide to Readers

This book results from the authors' experience and tries to address the widely acknowledged difficulty in communication between the experts in forensic genetics (FG) and laypersons. This communication gap is generally attributed to a supposed inherent difficulty of the scientific discipline but is also a result of the lack of experts' having consensual approaches on how to report the results of their analyses and the framing of their answers to the questions of interest.

The book was thus written having in mind not only law-related professionals, such as criminal investigators, mediators, lawyers, or judges, but also practitioners in laboratories performing genetic analyses and of course, self-learners enthusiastic about the discipline.

The main purpose is therefore to provide non-experts in genetics with the shortest possible text providing the correct interpretation of the forensic genetic reports for a wide range of problems, including both human and non-human analyses, without the need to attend a formal course on genetics and statistics.

It adopts a problem/example-based approach and the required background in genetics is presented as appendices, allowing the more inquisitive reader to access the theory and statistics behind each type of question and corresponding report.

The first chapter is dedicated to showing and typifying the multiple ways genetics can contribute to solving potential or formalized legal conflicts and to clarifying the differences between forensic genetics and the other sciences applied to the same issues, with a special emphasis on the (non) assumption of the discernible uniqueness principle.

The next chapters are devoted to the diverse types of legal issues and corresponding genetic approaches, including not only the 'classical' ones, using human DNA, but also those applied to non-human sources, from simple ancillary tools on criminalistics (silent witnesses) to food mislabeling or wildlife protected species.

Another critical point analyzed and debated throughout is the overlooked fact that different modes of genetic transmission do exist in the same species (humans possess three) and across distinct species, each of them with distinct possibilities and limitations in terms of probatory value.

Too frequently, FG is called "DNA", or "DNA analysis". This label not only undervalues the complexity of this branch of science but also forgets that DNA is not the only source of evidence in FG, an issue that is also addressed with examples of RNA virus and body fluids identification.

Finally, considering the target audience and objectives, despite the important role of genetics in the investigative phase it will not be discussed in depth here; instead, the focus will be on the production and reporting of court-admissible evidence. Therefore, the new and spectacular developments in genealogical forensics as investigative tools are just briefly presented as well as all their applications which may violate ethical or legal principles and regulations, compromising their admissibility as evidence in court. A discussion on the general ethical and legal issues pertaining to FG practices is however included.

The book is designed to be used and read in multiple ways: in the classical form, from start to end, and/or by consulting each type of question of interest (and the corresponding appendices, if needed, as well as the glossary). Using a literary metaphor, it can be read either as a novel, or a collection of interconnected short stories. In any case, the reading of both the first, introductory, chapter and the last one, is recommended: the first aims to provide means to understand and bypass the communication problems, and the last analyses state of the art FG, societal implications, and challenges.

Preface

The technological advancements in deciphering DNA sequence contents had a tremendous impact on many fields of pure and applied sciences. Forensic Genetics is one of them, and DNA based technologies have profoundly extended its power and significantly increased the amount of information provided to help justice enforcement, either by creating new ways of disclosing intelligence leads and providing novel evidentiary materials, or by magnifying the values of obtained quantifiable evidence.

Paradoxically, however, these advancements were accompanied by the belief that the sophistication and intricacies involved had turned the contribution of DNA impenetrable to non-experts, particularly when involving calculations pertaining to population genetics theory.

Our aim is to enable non-experts to understand the enormous potential of genetics in contributing to resolve litigations, either of civil or criminal nature. It is our experience that the main difficulties in the comprehension and (mis)use of Forensic Genetics derive from the poor communication between the geneticists and the users of the produced information (including not exclusively lawyers and judges), and do not arise primarily from a lack of knowledge of genetics.

We sustain that a simple and basic acquaintance with genetics theory is sufficient to ensure a successful and correct use of such results in the forensic context, or at least to minimize the degree of misunderstandings and to prevent the blind and irresponsible acceptance of DNA based evidentiary reports.

Deeply trusting that non-experts can grasp the essentials required to critically address most of the experts' reports, this book tries to contribute to install this healthier situation. To the readers the judgement if our aim has been reached.

Acknowledgements

It is impossible to list all persons and institutions who have contributed to this work. Iva Gomes, who critically revised the organization of the book contents and drafted BOX 12 (Investigating the Type of Biological Sample) deserves however a special thanks.

The authors were partially financed by FEDER (Fundo Europeu de Desenvolvimento Regional) funds through the COMPETE 2020–Operacional Program for Competitiveness and Internationalization (POCI), Portugal 2020, and by Portuguese funds through Fundação para a Ciência e a Tecnologia (FCT)/Ministério da Ciência, Tecnologia e Inovação within the framework of the projects by the Institute for Research and Innovation in Health Sciences (POCI-01–0145-FEDER-007274). NP is supported by FCT (Ref. 2022.04997.CEECIND).

Contents

V. Annexes

Glossary

Allele – each of the alternative forms of materializing the genetic information at a locus; in terms of the material basis of the coding of genetic information, a difference in DNA sequence at a specific locus.

Autosome – a chromosome or locus which has the same number of copies (2) in both sexes (BOX 5).

Carrier – an individual who is heterozygous for a recessive allele.

Characteristic – synonym of 'trait'; see Mendelian characteristic.

Chain of custody - documentation recording the sequence of events vis-à-vis evidence collection and handling.

Chimera – an individual in which cell lines from two or more different zygotes are found (see mosaic; BOX 11).

Chromosome – each of the cell structures containing a unit of DNA (see BOX 5).

Clone – each of the individuals, or groups of cells, which descend from a common ancestor by means of asexual reproduction (BOX 1), so that their genetic makeup is the same, barring mutation.

Codominance – the relationship between alleles that allows, using the standard analysis, the distinction between all genotypes involving them. An example from ABO blood groups: A and B alleles are codominant and so AB phenotype informs that individuals of that blood group have genotype AB, while individuals A can be either AA or AO, and individuals B, either BB or BO, since allele O is recessive, that is, goes unnoticed if in presence of A or B; A and B are therefore codominant to each other, but both dominant over O.

Deoxyribonucleic acid – see DNA.

Diploid – see Ploidy.

Directed mutagenesis – (any method allowing) the design of specific mutations.

Dizygotic – twins who have resulted from two eggs.

DNA – acronym for deoxyribonucleic acid, the chemical species in which genetic information is encoded; it is transcribed into RNA which, in turn is translated into proteins. Some viruses use RNA as genetic material.

Dominance – an allele *A* is dominant relatively to another one, recessive, symbolized by *a*, if individuals classified into phenotype A with standard methods can be either AA or Aa (see Codominance).

Egg – same as zygote, the fusion of a sperm and an egg (see BOX 1).

Exclusion – see BOX 17.

Gene – synonym of locus or allele, depending on context.

Gene editing – a group of technologies allowing genetic material to be added, removed, or altered, at specific locations in the genome.

Genetic profile – when applied to an individual, the description of its genotypes at the examined loci; at the population level, the array of allele frequencies at the studied loci.

Genetically modified organism (GMO) – an organism, with the exception of human beings, in which the genetic material has been altered in a way that does not occur naturally by mating and/or natural recombination (defined according to EU regulations: EUR-Lex – l28130 – EN – EUR-Lex (europa.eu), CONSULTED 28/12/2021); see also BOX 19.

Genome – the full set of genetic information of a system (an individual, a cell, etc.).

Genotype – each of the classes into which the individuals of a population can be grouped, according to the allelic state of the locus under study. For the standard mode of transmission, in each individual, it is composed of two alleles, identical or not, per individual. In the case of being identical, the individual is said to be a homozygote, whereas it is called heterozygote in the other case.

Germinal mutation – any hereditary alteration in the contents or structure of the genetic material transmitted to individual offspring (see BOXES 1 and 10). Usually referred to simply as mutation (see somatic mutation).

GMO – see 'Genetically Modified Organism'.

Haploid – see 'Ploidy'.

Heteroplasmy – the presence of more than one type of mtDNA in the same cell or organism (it can also apply to plastid DNA; BOX 1).

Heterozygosity – the state of a locus containing two different alleles; see 'Genotype'.

Heterozygote – an individual who is heterozygous at the locus under analysis; see 'Genotype'.

Heterozygous – same as 'Heterozygote'.

Homozygosity – the state of a locus containing two identical alleles; see 'Genotype'.

Homozygote – an individual who is homozygous at the locus under analysis; see 'Genotype'.

Homozygous – same as 'Homozygote'.

Likelihood ratio – The fraction in which the numerator is the probability of an event under a certain hypothesis and the denominator the probability of the same event assuming an alternative explanation (BOX 14).

Locus (plural: loci) – level of genetic information corresponding to a Mendelian characteristic; a specific position at the genome.

Mendelian characteristic – observation unit that presents, in the population under study, a discontinuous distribution (the individuals appear grouped into classes or types) and for which a simple mode of transmission is established. Examples: ABO and Rhesus blood groups.

Mendelian theory of heredity - (applied to the standard transmission mode) states that for each Mendelian phenotype, two alleles exist per locus per individual (one of maternal origin, another paternal) but just one of them is transmitted to offspring, the choice being random (i.e., the probability of each type is ½).

Mitochondrial DNA – see mtDNA.

Monozygotic – twins (or higher order multiple births) who have resulted from a single egg.

Mosaic – an individual comprising cells with different genetic composition resulting from somatic mutation occurring in the division of a single zygote (see chimera; BOX 11).

mtDNA – acronym for mitochondrial DNA, a part of our genome only transmitted maternally (see BOX 1).

Mutation – any hereditary alteration in the contents or structure of the genetic material (see BOXES 1 and 10). Usually employed in the sense of germinal, but can also be somatic.

Null – a synonym for 'silent (preferred in forensics) allele'.

PCR – the acronym for 'Polymerase Chain Reaction', a technique used to increase the quantity of genetic material present in a sample, in order to obtain enough DNA copies for subsequent analyses (see BOX 13).

Phenotype – each of the classes into which the individuals of a population can be grouped according to a Mendelian characteristic. Example: blood type A in ABO system.

Ploidy – number of copies of homologous genetic information present in a cell. Normal body cells contain two copies of each autosomal chromosome and thus are said diploid. Gametes (sperm or ovum) contain only one and are thus haploid.

Polymerase Chain Reaction – see 'PCR'.

Protein – a chemical type composed by units (a polymer of amino acids); for each protein, the sequential specification of the composing units and its length are encoded, at the DNA level in the corresponding locus. As a rule, to each locus corresponds one protein. Chemically, proteins are the structural and functional basis of living beings, and thus can be regarded as a kind of first level phenotype.

Recessive – an allele is recessive relatively to another if its presence in an individual can go unnoticed when in presence of a dominant (see 'Codominance').

Ribonucleic acid – see 'RNA'.

RNA – acronym for ribonucleic acid (see 'DNA').

Silent – a rare allele that goes undetected by standard analysis (see 'recessiveness').

Somatic mutation – any mutation occurring during the development of an individual's body, but not involving the reproductive cells and therefore not transmitted to offspring (see 'germinal mutation' and BOXES 1 and 10).

Trait – see 'characteristic'.

Transmission mode – not all genetic information is transmitted in the standard form (the one used preferentially in forensics) described by the Mendelian theory of heredity; some are sex-linked or sex-limited (see BOX 5).

Zygote – same as 'egg' (see BOX 1).

I
Introduction
Definitions and Framework

Introduction

The ambition of this book is to enable non-experts to understand and use the enormous potential of genetics (BOXes 2 to 5) to resolve litigations, either of a civil or criminal nature. Although its title, "Introduction to Forensic Genetics for Non-geneticists" may suggest that it comprises another course on forensic genetics (from now on, referred to as 'FG'), we aim to attain the formulated goal outside the learning approach and objectives of a classical course.

Indeed, it is our experience that the main difficulties in the comprehension and (mis)use of FG resides in communication between the geneticists and the diverse users of the produced information (including, among many others, lawyers and judges), and do not arise primarily from the lack of knowledge of genetics. It does not mean that genetics knowledge is irrelevant – on the contrary, it greatly enhances the proper forensic application of this branch of science. What we claim is simply that the acquaintance with genetics is by itself insufficient to ensure the successful and correct use of such results in a forensic context.

We have therefore approached an introduction to FG using a question-and-answer (Q&A) methodology, instead of providing a handbook that might miss its interfacial essence. We concretized this approach by typifying the questions that can be addressed by genetic expertise, presenting the essential biological and statistical genetics background to each topic being discussed in the form of boxes/appendices.

In Figure I.1, we try to provide a general overview of the kinds of problems approachable by FG, related Q&As chapters, as well as their classification into the broad types of perspective of their analysis.

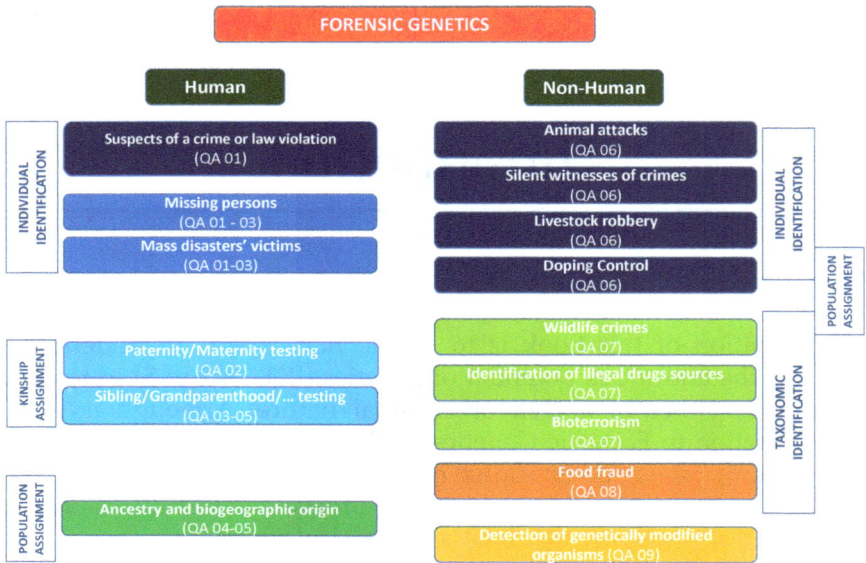

Figure I.1. Kinds of problems forensic genetics can help to solve. For each of them (in colored boxes), the corresponding Question & Answer (Q&A) book chapters are shown, and their integration into broad categories of theoretical approach is displayed (in vertical white boxes).

This approach does not prevent the analysis of the investigative facet of FG, as we will include 'open' questions and their role in the construction of leads and identification of suspects in the absence of any other non-genetic evidence. The Q&A approach is also appropriate for distinguishing the role of the FG expert from the one of police intelligence, which sometimes overlaps in the same person or institution, with the consequent and undesirable loss of independence.

At this point, and before undertaking the Q&As, it is necessary for the reader to understand: (i) that FG has a nature distinctive from that of other forensic sciences, (ii) which kinds of problems can (or cannot) be addressed by the FG, and (iii) that there is a double comprehension gap between users and experts: one residing in the translation of the forensic question in genetic terms and, symmetrically, another one in the conversion of the geneticist's report into forensically meaningful conclusions.

What is Forensic Genetics?

A widely accepted FG definition is the one presented at the launching of the first specially dedicated scientific journal (*Forensic Science International: Genetics*; https://www.journals.elsevier.com/forensic-science-international-genetics) to this branch of forensic science: "application of genetics to human and non-human material (in the sense of a science with the purpose of studying inherited characteristics for the analysis of inter- and intra-specific variations in populations) for the resolution of legal conflicts".

To this definition, we only dare to add that, besides the contribution to the resolution of legal conflicts, genetics has become increasingly interventive in the investigative phase of the criminal framework (namely, when helping to find a suspect in the absence of other, non-genetic, types of evidence) and also that it is increasingly used outside formal legal proceedings (for instance, settling doubtful paternities). This means that the actual role of FG greatly exceeds the classical one, that is, being used as an expert witness in court. In both cases, FG greatly contributes to alleviating the court trial's burden, either by helping with an extrajudicial arrangement or by ruling out inconsequent leads of suspicion. Indeed, classical paternity disputes are currently the vast majority of cases solved extrajudicially using the results of a genetic test, and prosecutors wait for the results of the genetic profiling of crime scene evidence before presenting (or not) a suspect.

The above definition, albeit correct, may be misleading as it can suggest that FG is just another forensic science, among many others. This is however not the case: FG is intrinsically different from 'classical' forensic sciences (CFSs), such as lophoscopy (fingerprint analysis) or ballistics, and this is reflected in the ways the expertise is framed and conducted, as well as in the resulting information presented. CFSs assume the *discernible uniqueness* principle, which states that markings or traces produced or left behind by different people or objects are observably different. Consequently, when two markings are not observably distinct, CFSs experts infer that they were made by the same person or object, and, conversely, if the expert deems the traces as different, the categorical conclusion is that they have different origins. For example, two distinguishable fingerprints imply two individuals, and conversely, two indistinguishable fingerprints imply the same individual. On the contrary, *FG works with types* (e.g., genotypes ↑Glossary) and therefore *all individuals belonging to the same class are indistinguishable*. The principle is the same as for the ABO blood groups, for example, in which case, two individuals with blood type AB are indistinguishable.

On the other hand, FG is able to compute *expected frequencies of observations under forensically relevant alternative scenarios*, based on population genetics theory (↑BOX 8) and statistical estimation of parameters (↑BOX 9). This opposition is summarized in Table I.1.

Table I.1. Epistemological distinction between forensic genetics and the other forensic sciences.

'CLASSICAL' FORENSIC SCIENCES (CFS)	FORENSIC GENETICS (FG)
Assume the discernible uniqueness principle *Ex: Each individual evidence corresponds to a specific, individual source.*	Does not depend on the discernible uniqueness assumption *Ex: Each individual evidence may be attributed to various individual sources.*
Aim at individualization *Ex: Every individual has a unique fingerprint.*	Aims at classification *Ex: Each individual is assigned to a type/ category (viz, blood group, genotype).*
Direct use of observations *Ex: Each observation is used as a whole, and every detail (qualitative or quantitative) counts.*	Uses types of observations (digital information) *Ex: The information from the evidence is processed in order to assign it to categories.*
Unable to calculate expected frequencies *Ex: Although sometimes using empirical estimates of the frequency of an evidence feature, it cannot predict the frequency of previously unobserved ones.*	Able to calculate expected values *Ex: Although using empirical estimates those are grounded in a theoretical framework, allowing to calculate expected frequencies, including for unobserved events.*

The consequences for the FG *modus operandi*, in contrast with CFSs, are that: (i) FG does not seek individualization, (ii) the results of FG expertise are expressed in terms of a comparison between expected frequencies of a genetic profile under alternative explanations for its occurrence (some limitations may, however, apply to cases of non-human materials, as will be discussed next in Chapters II.6 to II.9), and (iii) there is less room for expert opinion, the importance of his/her experience being comparatively minor. In fact, experts' education and training remain technically relevant, particularly in the treatment and interpretation of raw observational data. These contrasts are summarized and illustrated in Table I.2.

Table I.2. Operational distinction between forensic genetics and the other forensic sciences. An example contrasting the classical fingerprint analysis with genetics.

'CLASSICAL' FORENSIC SCIENCES (CFS)	FORENSIC GENETICS (FG)
Two fingerprints— one from the suspect and another from the crime scene—are considered as identical.	Two samples—one from the suspect and another from the crime scene—are of the same group/type.
Expert conclusion: They are from the same individual.	Expert conclusion: They are from the same individual *or* from distinct individuals, but of the same type.

A final word on the (mis)use of DNA (↑Glossary) analysis as an FG synonym: Not only does FG use other types of chemical substances as evidence (e.g., RNA ↑Glossary), referring to FG as 'DNA analysis' is also misleading in the sense that DNA analysis is just a small part of a process in which genetics theory and statistics also intervene.

What kind of problems can (or cannot) be answered by Forensic Genetics?

As FG does not individualize but just categorizes objects into types, individualization (as it would be desired in criminalistics or in a paternity investigation) is, in theoretical terms and by definition, impossible. It is however possible, for instance, in a paternity case in which both the alleged father and child are typed, to estimate the expected frequency of the genetic profile (↑Glossary) of the putative father assuming true paternity, as well as the expected frequency of the same profile under the hypothesis of the individuals being unrelated. In fact, and under some critical assumptions to be detailed below, the ratio between the two figures takes, using routinely employed analyses, astronomically large values, being erroneously taken by non experts as corresponding to individualization. This issue will be revisited in and materialized for each type of Q&A presented below.

Besides this basal problem, there are others depending on either biological or technical limitations. Among the first, true twinning is one of the most relevant: monozygotic twins are genetically very hard to distinguish, to say the least. The reasons behind this are the same that explain why distinct parts of the same individual body may exhibit different genetic profiles (but there are other explanations for this intraindividual genetic heterogeneity). The technical issues are multivariate but are particularly important in the cases of vestigial and/ or degraded samples, as is frequently the case in crime scene traces.

The comprehension gaps between users and experts

There is a double fold comprehension gap between users and geneticists: on the translation of the forensic question in genetic terms and, the other way around, in the conversion of the geneticist's report into a forensically meaningful conclusion.

The first gap is created by many factors, which include misunderstandings on (*i*) the distinctive nature of FG relative to CFSs, to which most non-experts are more familiar with, and (*ii*) on the role of the expert, both exacerbated by the so-called CSI effect (from the TV series Crime Scene Investigation). Indeed, the questions that a court would like to be answered are individual, as for instance, "Is the suspect the author of the crime?". Firstly, the FG expert cannot express any opinion on the *authorship* of a crime but simply on the *genetic origin* of certain biological material. That is – the presence of a trace at a crime scene is a piece of evidence (sometimes irrelevant, as when the suspect is/was frequently present at the crime scene, as a visitor or coinhabitant of a private home or a public place), but it does not imply a criminal behavior. This profound conceptual difference has been extensively analyzed and the results are summarized next.

Levels and hierarchy of propositions

Assertions on the causes or, in general, relations between phenomena or data obtained from observations are, in scientific parlance, called *hypotheses* (such as "AIDS is caused by a virus."). In forensics, the equivalent concept is also known as *propositions*. Let us suppose that in a criminal case both the suspect (John Doe) and the crime scene sample have revealed the same genetic profile. The ultimately relevant forensic question, "Is John Doe the author of the crime?" has two answers in the form of two alternative, mutually exclusive propositions: one from the accusation (e.g., "John Doe is the author of the crime"), and one from the defense ("The unknown author of the crime is someone else other than John Doe").

FG is unable to directly answer to these propositions: not only, as already evidenced, because FG does not provide individualization, but also because the propositions FG can indeed address are indirect and of a much lower – indeed, the lowest, level: "John Doe is the source of the crime scene sample" and the alternative "The source of the crime scene sample is an unknown individual, with the same genetic profile as John Doe". The full picture can be visualized in the scheme below (Table I.3):

Table 1.3. The levels of the hierarchy of propositions. A: Accusation; D: Defense; S: Suspect; V: Victim. Adapted from Gittelson et al., 2016.

Propositions		Description/Examples
Level	Type	
3	Offense	A: S purposedly beat V to death D: S and V had a fight; S had no killing intentions and just defended him/herself *NB: only relevant in criminal cases*
2	Activity	A: S and V had a fight D: S and V were playing a game
1	Source	A: Blood found at V's clothes is from S D: Blood found at V's clothes is from someone else
0	Sub-source	A: The genetic profile found at V's clothes is from S D: : The genetic profile found at V's clothes is from someone else

It is obvious that, strictly speaking, an expert in FG can only provide information at the sub-source level. Although significant progresses on the elucidation of the probable type of biological source involved (e.g., semen, blood, saliva, etc.) as addressed at level 1 (source level) have accumulated, the interpretation of these results requires knowledge that goes beyond genetic analysis proper (BOX 12).

Quantification of the probatory value of the evidence

We have seen that typical FG results of the analysis of any evidence do not provide individualization, but only classification, i.e., that the trace could be as well attributed to an individual or to anyone else sharing the same genetic profile (↑Glossary). This means that instead of individualization, we face an identification problem, that is, *contrarily to 'classical' forensic sciences approach, we do not assume that, since the two profiles are identical, it implies that they are unique and thus attributable to a single individual source.* It follows that quantifying the evidentiary value of these results is necessarily a comparative task: we must compare the chances of observing the obtained genetic results assuming each one of the two possibilities (established prior to any genetic analysis). These two possibilities correspond exactly to alternative propositions at the (sub)source level.

The identification problem can be formulated in a more general, neutral, form as: *given that two samples have revealed the same genetic profile*, what are the chances that (*i*) they have the same individual origin, or (*ii*) they are from different individuals? In the standard form,

H1: The source of the two samples is the same individual.

H2: The two samples are from different, unrelated, individuals.

The task of the FG expert is then to calculate the corresponding probabilities (or, better, the expected frequencies of the genetic profile, under the genetic theory), which is symbolized as

P(R|H1): The expected frequency of an individual with that profile in the population, that is, the probability of the result (R) assuming H1 (a single individual source); and

P(R|H2): The expected frequency of a pair of individuals with that profile in the population, that is, the probability of the result R assuming H2 (a dual individual source).

We can therefore compute the **ratio**:

$$LR = \frac{P(R|H1)}{P(R|H2)}$$

Obviously, P|H1 and P|H2 have different values. While the first is simply the frequency of the profile in the population (or the probability of finding, at random, in the population an individual with that profile), the second is the probability of finding, also at random, a pair of individuals with the same profile.

The expert would then report:

> *The genetic results are LR times more probable (likely, or frequent) under the hypothesis that they have a single individual source (H1), rather than having been originated from two distinct individuals (H2).*

Some considerations on this form of communication are essential before concluding:

1. LR is not a probability, but a **ratio** of probabilities. It means that it only makes sense in a comparative manner, rather than in an absolute form. Both the numerator and denominator are conditioned to the specified hypotheses; there could be other hypotheses to be considered, such as involving more individuals or being from two relatives, as full sibs, etc. (BOX 14).

2. The reported format assumes that H1 and H2 are mutually exclusive and exhaustive, that is, there was, per sample, a single contributor (no partial contributions or mixtures), and all other explanations for the sources of the samples considered excluded. Very importantly, there must be no evidence in the obtained results supporting the possibility of multiple contributors. When this condition is not met, a quite different, and both theoretically and technically much more difficult problem arises, namely, to establish if the suspect is possibly a contributor to the mixture, or, in other words, if the suspect's profile is probably contained in the complex profile (BOX 13).

3. A large, but variable number of extra assumptions from genetic theory and of statistical nature are used; they will be specified, as will their limiting effect on the conclusions when handling each type of problem in the section with Q&As.

FURTHER INFO

Amorim, A. and Budowle, B. (2016). Definition and purpose. pp. 1–12. *In*: Amorim, A. and Budowle, B. (eds.). Handbook of Forensic Genetics: Biodiversity and Heredity in Civil and Criminal Investigation. World Scientific, New Jersey. doi: 10.1142/q0023.

Biedermann, A. (2022). The strange persistence of (source) "identification" claims in forensic literature through descriptivism, diagnosticism and machinism. Forensic Science International: Synergy, 4: 100222. https://doi.org/10.1016/j.fsisyn.2022.100222.

Carlson, Laura, Kennedy, Jarrah, Zeller, Kimberly and Busey, Thomas. (2021). Describing communication during a forensic investigation using the pebbles on a Scale Metaphor. Forensic Science International: Synergy, 100199. 10.1016/j.fsisyn.2021.100199.

Costa, S. (2022). DNA as 'ready-made evidence': An analysis of Portuguese judges' views. The International Journal of Evidence & Proof., 26(2): 121–135. doi:10.1177/13657127211070331.

Crispino, F., Weyermann, C., Delémont, O., Roux, C. and Ribaux, O. (2022). Towards another paradigm for forensic science? WIREs Forensic Science, 4(3): e1441. https://doi.org/10.1002/wfs2.1441.

David, H. and Kaye, D.H. (2010). Probability, Individualization, and Uniqueness in Forensic Science Evidence: Listening to the Academies. Brooklyn Law Review, 75 Brook. L. Rev., 75: 1163.

David, H. Kaye. (2010). Probability, Individualization, and Uniqueness in Forensic Science Evidence: Listening to the Academies, 75 Brook. L. Rev., 1163.

David, H. Kaye. (2010). Probability, Individualization, and Uniqueness in Forensic Science Evidence: Listening to the Academies, 75 Brook. L. Rev., 1163.

Errickson, D., Giles, S.B. and Horsman, G. (2019). The CSI Effect (s no one?). J. Forensic Leg. Med., 67: 64-65. doi: 10.1016/j.jflm.2019.05.017.

Gill, P., Hicks, T., Butler, J.M., Connolly, E., Gusmão, L., Kokshoorn, B., Morling, N., van Oorschot, R.A.H., Parson, W., Prinz, M., Schneider, P.M., Sijen, T. and Taylor, D. (2018). DNA commission of the International society for forensic genetics: Assessing the value of forensic biological evidence—Guidelines highlighting the importance of propositions: Part I: evaluation of DNA profiling comparisons given (sub-) source propositions. Forensic Sci. Int. Genet., 36: 189–202. doi: 10.1016/j.fsigen.2018.07.003.

Gittelson, S., Kalafut, T., Myers, S., Taylor, D., Hicks, T., Taroni, F., Evett, I.W., Bright, J.A. and Buckleton, J. (2016). A practical guide for the formulation of propositions in the bayesian approach to DNA evidence interpretation in an adversarial environment. J. Forensic Sci., 61(1): 186-95. doi: 10.1111/1556-4029.12907.

Heavey, A.L., Turbett, G.R., Houck, M.M. and Lewis, S.W. (2021). Toward a common language for quality issues in forensic science. Wiley Interdisciplinary Reviews: Forensic Science, e1452. https://doi.org/10.1002/wfs2.1452.

Hicks, T., Buckleton, J., Castella, V., Evett, I. and Jackson, G. (2022). A logical framework for forensic DNA interpretation. Genes, 13(6): 957. https://doi.org/10.3390/genes13060957.

Jason, M. Chin and Carlos, M. Ibaviosa. (2022). Beyond CSI: Calibrating public beliefs about the reliability of forensic science through openness and transparency. Science & Justice, 62(3): 272–283. https://doi.org/10.1016/j.scijus.2022.02.006.

Lindsey, Samuel, Hertwig, Ralph and Gigerenzer, Gerd. (2003). Communicating statistical DNA evidence. Jurimetrics, 43: 147–163.

Ribeiro, G., Tangen, J.M. and McKimmie, B.M. (2019). Beliefs about error rates and human judgment in forensic science. Forensic Sci. Int., 297: 138–147. doi: 10.1016/j.forsciint.2019.01.034.

Saks, M.J. and Koehler, J.J. (2005). The coming paradigm shift in forensic identification. Science, 309: 892–895.

Spellman, B.A., Eldridge, H. and Bieber, P. (2021). Challenges to reasoning in forensic science decisions. Forensic Science International: Synergy, 100200. https://doi.org/10.1016/j.fsisyn.2021.100200.

Thompson, W.C., Vuille, J., Taroni, F. and Biedermann, A. (2018). After uniqueness: The evolution of forensic science opinions. Judicature, 102(1): 18–27.

Valerio, R. (2020). Likelihood ratios for lawyers…I didn't go to law school for this! WIREs Forensic Sci., 2: e1366. https://doi.org/10.1002/wfs2.1366.

Yoon, J.Y., Prinz, M., McKiernan, H. and Oldoni, F. (2022). American forensic DNA practitioners' opinion on activity level evaluative reporting. J. Forensic Sci., 00: 1–13. https://doi.org/10.1111/1556-4029.15063.

II
Questions & Answers

Introduction

In this section, we will analyze the different types of (at least potentially) forensically relevant questions that are already routinely answered by FG (Forensic Genetics). For each situation, the entire flow of information is mapped, the crucial steps are described in detail, as well as the way FG addresses the case, assumptions, and difficulties involved. The genetics theory and techniques employed are deferred to in the explanatory appendices. We adopted a general formal scheme that fits both investigative and probatory situations. The general flowchart is as follows:

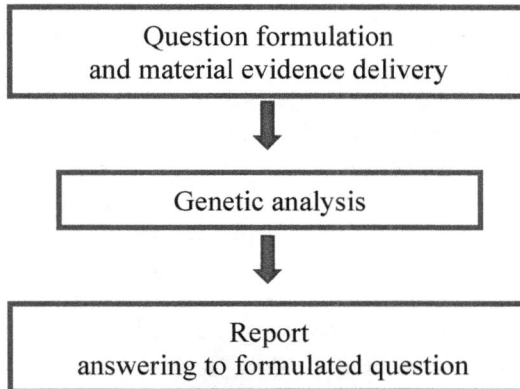

```
┌─────────────────────────────────────┐
│       Question formulation            │
│  and material evidence delivery       │
└─────────────────────────────────────┘
                  ↓
     ┌───────────────────────────┐
     │      Genetic analysis      │
     └───────────────────────────┘
                  ↓
┌─────────────────────────────────────┐
│             Report                    │
│   answering to formulated question    │
└─────────────────────────────────────┘
```

As previously explained this simple, unidirectional scheme is often recursive, due to interactions between the experts and the requesting parties. This happens namely in cases for which the formulated question raises doubts, as well as when collection details, and more, or larger quantities of, evidentiary items are asked for.

1. Human identification: *Is this trace from John Doe?*

The quintessential question in criminalistics, although not restricted to criminal proceedings is: who committed the crime (or, more generally, who performed a certain action)? To allow the contribution of Forensic Genetics (FG) to answer these questions, it is necessary to obtain some material found at the crime scene – or in any case undisputedly associated with the criminal activity – which can be used to trace the author(s) of the crime. In this section, we will discuss the question of identification in the framework of criminal investigation, using the terminology of this context: "traces" or "stains" for the biological sample recovered from the crime scene for which donors are sought, and "suspect" for the reference individual who will be analyzed as a possible donor of the sample. It must be stressed that the same formal approach is used for any personal identification, namely in the identification of corpses (or body parts), involved or not in mass disasters, with the appropriate terminological changes. For example, the comparison between the genetic profile recovered from a missing person's toothbrush and the one obtained from a human corpse found near his/her home.

Traces of saliva or other biological fluid, hairs, dandruff, or even material left by contact on objects' surfaces, such as cigarette butts, drinking glasses, and so on, frequently take the vestigial form. This fact leaves plenty of room for pitfalls in their genetic analyses, as they are of vestigial quantities, often degraded and, worse still, contaminated (i.e., containing genetic material from various contributors, sometimes the collectors themselves). These problems can seriously compromise the contribution of FG in helping to solve the crime and are the object of intense research (BOX 13). In the following section, we will assume that the material evidence to be genetically analyzed is genuine, uncontaminated (has a single source), and presented in sufficient amount and good preservation conditions, but we will return to the discussion of these problems when concluding the section.

The next steps depend on the existence (1.a) or not (1.b) of a suspect (person of interest, missing individual) whose genetic profile (↑Glossary) is known or obtainable during the investigation. The first section is therefore associated with the evaluation of evidence ('proof context') while the second is described as it happens in the investigative phase. Ideally, if the latter approach is successful, it provides evidence to substantiate the first one.

1.a. *Comparison of genetic profiles between trace and suspect*

Assuming that all the above conditions are met, it is then possible to compare the single source genetic profile found in the vestige with the one from the suspect. These samples can be both analyzed during the case or by using a previously typed profile of a suspect, which may be deposited in a forensic DNA database (BOX 15) or, as in non-criminal cases, other repositories, as those used to get insights on genetic ancestry or predispositions to diseases.

The result of the comparison between the profiles of the vestige and the suspect may be that either the two are identical for all the genetic markers (↑Glossary) or otherwise. In the first case, the likelihood of the event will be reported in the form of a ratio, in which:

- the numerator is the expected frequency (BOX 8) of the profile in the relevant population under the main hypothesis (H1) that they are from the same individual, and
- the denominator is the expected frequency of the same profile being observed in a random pair of individuals in the relevant population, assuming the alternative hypothesis (H2), that the suspect and crime scene sample donor are distinct, unrelated, individuals randomly sampled in the relevant population.

The first is symbolized as P(O|H1) (read as "probability of the observation given, or assuming, H1"), and the second is accordingly symbolized as P(O|H2).

Then, the obtained result will be reported through what is usually called the **likelihood ratio (LR)** (BOX 14),

$$LR = P(O|H1)/P(O|H2),$$

which can be phrased as "the genetic results obtained are expected to be observed LR times more frequently, assuming the crime scene sample is from the suspect than assuming it came from another, genetically unrelated, individual". It is noteworthy that LR may reach several orders of magnitude (> 10^{20}, e.g.) providing a very powerful statistical support for the suspect coinciding with the donor of the vestige sample.

Note that LR is *not* a probability, although it can be converted into one. This conversion is however debatable, as it requires more assumptions and involves the unnecessary risk of disturbing the independence of the expert when formulating prior probabilities.

The result of the comparison between the single source genetic profile found in the vestige and the one from the suspect may however be that the two profiles are not identical. It would seem at first sight that a categorical conclusion is possible in this situation: that the two profiles have certainly different donors, and therefore, the suspect is exonerated. The situation is not so simple, as it has been observed, albeit rarely, that different samples from the same donor may reveal distinct genetic profiles (BOX 11). Such a paradoxical situation, in which different parts of an individual body exhibit different genetic profiles, may be due to two types of causes. One is due to DNA replication errors (BOX 10) in his/her body (somatic mutation ↑Glossary) leading to mosaicism (↑Glossary). The second is called chimerism (↑Glossary) and occurs when the person's body contains parts from genetically distinct sources (caused, for instance, among other causes by transplantation or blood transfusion).

The solution to this conundrum is different in the two situations that, fortunately, are easily distinguishable reinspecting the differences observed between the profiles. Indeed, if we are in the presence of mosaicism, it is expected that the differences are minor (i.e., in a single or very few of the markers of the genetic profile), while in the case of chimerism a large number of differences is expected. To rule out chimerism as an explanation, the expert must check if (a) the suspect has received a transfusion or transplantation, and/or (b) if both the samples from the suspect and crime scene are originated from distinct body parts or fluids, asking, if possible, for the resampling of the suspect. The outcome of this extended investigation can reveal, however, that we are in the presence of a chimaera. For instance, it may happen that the profile found in the suspect's saliva and used as a reference sample, is different from the one obtained in the blood (due to a bone marrow transplantation, e.g.). It can then occur that the latter sample is identical to the one typed in the bloodstain found at the crime scene, contrarily to the first, obtained from saliva. In this case, a new hypothesis may arise: the donor of the crime scene stain could be, other than the suspect, the bone marrow donor.

On the other hand, if mosaicism is admitted as an explanation for the (few) differences between the profiles, the numerator of the ratio above must be generalized to incorporate this possibility, i.e., the occurrence of mutation(s). The way to do it is however still not consensual and the relative rarity of these cases explains the difficulty in estimating the frequency of the phenomenon.

1.b. *Identification in the absence of a suspect*

This situation in criminalistics corresponds to cases in which non-genetic evidence is unable to guide the investigation in finding a suspect. One or more crime scene samples, however, can be successfully typed and produce unambiguous genetic profiles. For simplification, let us assume that a single profile is retrieved from the crime scene, but no suspect's profile is available for comparison. The same situation is sometimes found in cases of unidentified bodies (or parts of) for which there is, at the beginning of the investigation, no report of disappearance plausibly matching the circumstances of the case.

In criminalistics, a possible way to get around the impasse is to use a forensic DNA database (BOX 15) and to search for the presence of an identical, identified profile. If a match is found, this may equate to finding a suspect and proceeding with the investigation narrowed to him/her, depending however on the country's legal framework. From the FG point of view, it means that we will be in the situation we have dealt with in the previous section (1.a). It may happen that the databased profile contains a different set of markers from the one of the traces, but a good degree of overlapping is assumed, so that the number of markers common to both may be satisfactory to proceed with the identification of the suspect.

21

In some cases, however, the match is found to an unidentified stored profile (obtained from one or more other crime scene samples). Then, two or more independent investigations may now be focused on a single suspect, although unknown, by linking crimes thought to have been committed by different individuals and thus powerfully contribute to a successful identification and to solve various crimes.

When no exact match is found, some countries allow the querying of the database using what is called familial searching (BOX 15). In this procedure, near matches (that is, profiles that differ from the one retrieved from the crime scene in just one or a few markers) are investigated, assuming that the genetic similarity indicates they belong to close relatives of the perpetrator. For example, if complete hits are found in some markers, while in others the hits are incomplete or inexistent, the suspect may be a full sibling of the individual whose genetic profile is databased. On the other hand, if there are only partial or total hits for all the markers, the suspect may be a parent or an offspring of the databased individual. This procedure has led to mediatic, and spectacular solving of cases thought to be irresoluble or even closed. Of course, the more distant the relationships, the less likely is this correlation between the databased profile and the sought individual.

2. First-degree kinship (paternity/maternity): *Is John Doe the father of Ken?*

Among the first recorded contributions of genetics to forensic matters are paternity investigations, which still constitute a large fraction of routine work, both in public institutions and private laboratories. In the civil framework, paternity is by far the type of kinship most questioned, much more than maternity—the other first-degree relationship—due to the peculiar mammalian viviparous type of human reproduction (BOX 1). In criminalistics, paternity investigations usually emerge in cases related to sexual offenses, but other applications may arise, as in the case of missing persons, or disaster victims' identification. It must be said, that in the last two cases, whenever there is such an option, maternity investigation is preferred over paternity, due to the higher level of confidence in the parental relationship, the same happening in the situation of suspected exchange of babies, for example.

Since the standard approach is to consider the autosomal mode of genetic transmission (BOX 5), which implies that the markers analyzed are not sex-linked (BOX 3), paternity and maternity investigations are treated equally, whatever the sex of the offspring. That is, both technical and statistical procedures are the same for paternity and maternity cases, regardless if daughters or sons are involved. Therefore, in this section, we will use paternity examples, but the reader should be aware that the whole of what is written below applies also to maternity. In addition, for simplicity's sake, we will consider the context of a typical paternity test, where both the alleged father and the child are available for analysis, with no identification purposes. The alleged father is assumed (a) to not have any monozygotic twin, and (b) to be unrelated to the mother of the child. In the first case, as monozygotic twins expectedly share the same genetic information for the analyzed markers, the obtained results apply to any of the brothers. Thus, if a man with a monozygotic twin is analyzed as the alleged father in a paternity test, non-genetic evidence must be used to clarify who is indeed the real father of the child. If such non-genetic evidence is inexistent, the analysis of the genetic data may be fruitless or very complex, as it relies on the occurrence of somatic mutations (↑Glossary, BOX 11). On the other hand, if the alleged father is a close relative of the mother, a more complex framework to tackle the incestuous problem is required to weigh the genetic evidence, but powerful statistical results may anyhow be reached depending on the alternative kinship hypothesis and the genotypic configuration of the individuals.

There can be considered two situations in a paternity test, depending on the availability of the genetic profile (↑Glossary) of the other (undoubted) progenitor (the undoubted mother in paternity cases). We will consider them by order of simplicity, beginning with the duo case, where only the alleged father and the offspring are analyzed. We will then proceed to the case where a trio: alleged father, (undoubted) mother, and offspring are analyzed. In any case, it is noteworthy that we assume the standard propositions: the alleged father is either (a) truly the father or (b) unrelated to the real one. If, for instance, there is the possibility of the true father being a brother of the real one (i.e., the analyzed putative father may be an uncle of the offspring), this information should be available to the expert, as it changes the hypotheses at stake and significantly alters the calculations. The same happens if the assumption that the alleged father and the mother are unrelated is not met, as previously referred.

2.a. *Questioned father/offspring duo ('motherless case')*

We assume that we type, or have access to, the genetic profiles of both the putative father (PF) and the offspring (O), and the question is made as: is PF the biological father of O?

According to the previously outlined (Q &A I), we must proceed by calculating a likelihood ratio in which the numerator will be the expected frequency of this pair of genetic profiles assuming that (**H1**) PF and O are, indeed, biologically related as father and son/daughter. This is quite easily made (BOX 14) and the result is symbolized as P(R|H1). For the denominator, we need an alternative hypothesis, **H2**, which is generally not formulated by the requesting parties. From the genetic point of view, to formulate H2 as "PF is not the biological father of O" is insufficient, since not being the father, PF can be otherwise genetically related to O, for instance, as an uncle or grandfather. As previously referred to, these possibilities can also be incorporated as alternative hypotheses in the calculations but must be explicitly defined prior to any genetic analysis. In the most common situation, the alleged father and the offspring are alternatively assumed to be unrelated and thus **H2** is formulated as: PF is genetically unrelated to O (or PF was randomly chosen from the population). Similarly, the denominator is symbolized as $P(R|H2)$, and the likelihood ratio (often called *paternity index*) is now easily calculated as (BOX 14):

$$LR = P(R|H1)/P(R|H2).$$

The results can be phrased as:

> *The genetic observations are LR times more probable assuming that PF is the biological father of O than assuming they are unrelated.*

As previously in Q&A 1, the LR value may reach several orders of magnitude ($> 10^{15}$ or alternatively $< 10^{-15}$, e.g.), providing strong statistical support to one of the hypotheses at stake (paternity and unrelatedness, respectively). For each of the analyzed markers, the hypothesis H1, paternity, is typically favored when at least a partial match is obtained, that is, if at least one of the paternal alleles (↑Glossary) are shared with the offspring. If this match is observed for all the markers, the paternity hypothesis is expected to be strongly favored.

Rooted in the old Latin saying, *pater semper incertus est* (father is always uncertain), and in an erroneous use of the concept of 'exclusion' (BOX 17), a still frequent—and incorrect— way of approaching paternity investigation persists, however. In this approach, when incompatibilities with the genetic theory of Mendelian transmission are observed, that is, none of the paternal alleles are observed in the offspring, the categorical conclusion of paternity exclusion is reported. It is mandatory to state boldly that this approach is falsely grounded, since exceptions to the regular transmission rules, although rare, do exist. As we are facing a disputed paternity, it is grossly incorrect to assume that an incompatibility means the exclusion of paternity, when indeed, we may be in the presence of a true biological kinship, but in which a DNA copy error has occurred (in this case, a germinal mutation ↑Glossary) or a silent allele (↑Glossary) is present.

The incorporation of this possibility in the likelihood ratio is the correct approach allowing the report of the quantitative evaluation of the genetic evidence (BOXes 14 and 17). In this likelihood ratio, the probabilities associated with the (rare) phenomena referred to above (mutations and silent alleles) are considered. It should be however clear that the probability of an alleged father/offspring pair does not share genetic information in several markers due to mutations or silent alleles, instead of non-paternity, is virtually zero, if the number of analyzed markers increases. In any case, dedicated software can weigh the likelihood of the genotypic configurations, under the hypotheses in analysis and considering such complicating factors. This situation is extendable to the case when the undoubted parent of the child (typically the mother) is analyzed, as explained next.

2.b. *Questioned father/offspring kinship with mother's profile available*

In this situation, we have access to the genetic profiles of the putative father (PF) and the offspring (O), as well as the one from the unquestioned mother (M) of O. The question we are asked, is the same as above: is PF the biological father of O? The difference to the previous problem 2.a. is that, in this case, the specific paternal genetic information may be identified, given the maternal genetic information, which is now known.

As previously, to answer the question we must proceed by calculating a ratio in which the numerator is the expected frequency of this trio of genetic profiles assuming (H1) they are, biologically, related as a father (PF), mother (M), and son/daughter (O). This is quite simply performed (BOX 14) and the result is symbolized as P(R|H1). To calculate the denominator, an alternative hypothesis must be established, **H2**, which is again generally not formulated by the requesting parties. As above, to formulate H2 as "PF is not the biological father of O" is insufficient; not being the father, PF can be otherwise genetically related to O, and as before, it is traditional to assume they are unrelated. **H2** is now formulated as: PF is genetically unrelated to O, son/daughter of M (or he was chosen genetically at random). The denominator is now easily calculated (BOX 14) as: $P(R|H2)$, and the ratio will be

$$LR = P(R|H1)/P(R|H2),$$

which can be phrased as:

The genetic observations are LR times more probable assuming that PF is the biological father of O, undisputed son/daughter of M, than assuming they are unrelated.

It must be noted that the inclusion of the profile of M, although genetically informative, brings some problems which are absent in the "motherless cases". Indeed, the presented mother may be biologically false (e.g., due to a swap of babies at the hospital). This may be a rare and easily detected situation, but if occurs, introduces a serious ethical and deontological problem: can the expert report on something he/she was not asked for? On the other hand, if incompatibilities are showing up when considering the trio as biologically true (the offspring must exhibit one allele from the father and one from the mother), it is incorrect to assume they have a paternal origin, as mutations can also occur in mothers.

So, as in the motherless cases, the report must incorporate all the possibilities, both for paternal and maternal genetic transmission (BOX 17). In any case, the consideration of the mother generally improves the power of the calculations and results, compared with the situation where only the alleged father and the offspring are analyzed.

3. Other kinships: *Are John and Bill related as, for instance, sibs?*

The investigation of kinships more removed than identity and paternity/ maternity is, expectedly, more complex. This higher level of intricacy is due not only to its more demanding statistical and computational treatment but also to the corresponding interpretation of the results. Given this, problems related to kinships beyond identity (Q&A 01), or paternity/maternity (Q&A 02) are then known as "complex kinship problems".

These problems arise in a plethora of cases related to criminalistics, victims' identification, or civil litigations. In criminalistics, the question may arise for instance in a situation in which a profile recovered from a crime scene, possibly from the perpetrator, partially overlaps one found in a database when performing a familial search (Q&A 01 and BOX 15). Thus, if John's profile is stored in a DNA database and it partially matches with the one recovered from the crime scene (whose donor is Bill, let's say), FG experts may want to weigh the likelihood of a John's sibling being the donor sought. In victim identification problems, the approach is similar—if Bill, recognized as John's brother, is missing and an unidentified part of a body is found, FG experts may quantify the likelihood of it belonging to John's brother. In this case, the genetic profile of John would be compared with the one obtained from the found body's part. In the framework of civil cases, complex kinships may be analyzed as proxies of paternity investigations when the alleged father is not available for testing. Cases involving disputed heritages, in which a legally recognized offspring and/or other relatives are compared with an individual also claiming to be a relative of the deceased, are particularly common. The way the weight of the evidence is statistically computed is addressed in BOXes 7, 9, and 14.

At this point, it should be highlighted, especially for the cases of victim's identification or kinship assessment in which the questioned individual or the alleged parent(s) are not directly available for testing, that the statistical analyses are based on the assumption that the legal relationships between the individuals recruited for the analyses correspond to the genetic ones. For example, consider a situation where John claims the paternity of a deceased man, Bill. As the legally recognized son of Bill, Bill Jr is alive, a logical step may be to compare John's and Bill Jr's genetic profiles and then to quantify the likelihood of them being related as paternal half-brothers. Then, a statistical result favoring the alternative hypothesis (the individuals being unrelated) can be explained, not only because John is not a son of Bill, but also because the assumed son, Bill Jr, is not (and then it could happen that John is truly Bill's biological son!).

Other complexities are typically inherent to this type of problems, such as *(i)* the high number of individuals involved, *(ii)* the multiple alternative kinship hypotheses, or even *(iii)* the existence of hypotheses theoretically undistinguishable between them (at least when using the markers routinely used in FG). Indeed, if two or three samples and/or individuals are typically analyzed in identification and paternity/maternity problems, this number may increase when other relationships are at stake. A typical case of *(ii)* occurs when the simultaneous evaluation of the likelihood of two (or more) persons being related as full-sibs, half-sibs, or unrelated, is requested. Finally, the latter situation *(iii)* happens with some distinct kinships being undistinguishable when using unlinked markers with a specific mode of transmission (BOX 7). For example, considering a pair of individuals and unlinked autosomal markers, the pedigrees—half-siblings, grandparent-grandchild, and avuncular— are theoretically indistinguishable, such as the pedigrees: paternal half-sisters and mother-daughter, when unlinked X chromosome markers are analyzed (↑Glossary, BOX 5). Indeed, when using exclusively genetic information, two pedigrees may be theoretically indistinguishable regardless of the number of markers analyzed. A practical implication of this may arise, for example, if John claims that his father is either the father or the brother of Bill, John and Bill being thus either related as half-siblings or as avuncular, respectively. The hypotheses may have been formulated by John's representing parties considering what John's mother, who had been a young maid at Bill's family home, told him before dying. If only Bill and John are available for testing, it is useless to analyze their genetic profiles just with the standard unlinked autosomal markers, as it is *a priori* known that both hypotheses will be equally likely.

Here it must be highlighted that using markers with different modes of genetic transmission may help to disentangle the pedigrees of interest in a specific context (BOX 5). For example, if John and Bill were females, X chromosome markers will allow for weighing differently the abovementioned kinship hypotheses (paternal half-sisters vs. paternal aunt-niece). In the case of males, these markers would also be useless as autosomes, since their transmission is broken at any father-son transmission, equating both pedigrees: paternal half-brothers and the paternal uncle-nephew, to unrelated males. Notwithstanding, in this case, Y chromosomal markers would help to determine if Bill and John belong to the same paternal lineage (paternally related vs. unrelated), but the distinction between pedigrees (paternal half-brothers vs. uncle-nephew) would not be obtained.

Furthermore, pedigrees to be analyzed must be unambiguously defined and both geneticists and laypersons must be aware that everyday language may not be precise enough to establish genetic relationships (BOXes 6 and 7). For example, a pair of first cousins males, sons of two full-sisters, may share familial X chromosomal alleles, but not Y ones; contrary to the offspring of two full-brothers, which share familial Y chromosomal alleles but not X ones. Two male first cousins, offspring of a full-brother-sister pair, may only share familial autosomal alleles (BOX 7). Indeed, a pair of first cousins may be more or less related depending on the sex of the individuals and of the individuals linking them, as well as on the mode of genetic transmission considered.

With these precautions in mind, we will then proceed to examine two examples regarding sibship problems.

3.a. Are John and Bill full brothers?

Having both parents in common, a pair of full siblings may share both the paternal and maternal genetic inheritance, but they can also share just either the maternal or the paternal one, or even none of them. Indeed, for a diploid (↑Glossary) marker, a pair of full siblings share both the paternal and maternal genetic information (as monozygotic twins always do) with only 25% of probability. Analogously, the probability of not sharing neither the paternal nor the maternal genetic information (as unrelated individuals) is also 25%, while the probability of sharing exactly a half of the genetic information with common ancestry (as parent-child pairs) amounts to 50%. For the other modes of genetic transmission, the genetic proximity depends on the sex of the individuals (as previously explained with the example of first cousins). In the specific case of a pair of full brothers (as may be with John and Bill), the sharing of familial Y chromosomal genetic information occurs with 100% of probability, unless mutation occurs, dropping this probability to 50% in the case of X chromosomal markers.

It is expected that the set of autosomal markers standardly used in forensic routine may provide a statistically strong result when the hypothesis of Bill and John being related as full brothers is compared with the alternative one of being unrelated. Anyhow, the analysis of Y chromosomal patrilineage markers may provide strong evidence favoring the hypothesis of unrelatedness when the genetic profiles do not match. Conversely, in the case of matching, caution vis-à-vis the interpretation of the results should be taken, as matching would occur with all males paternally related, and not necessarily indicate full-sibship (see Q &A 5 and 6).

A quite different situation concerning the probative power of genetic analyses may be expected if the alternative hypothesis is John and Bill being half-brothers, instead of being unrelated. In this case, it is required to specify if the common ancestry is either paternal or maternal. Indeed, it is particularly common the situation in which siblings do not doubt the common maternity, contrarily to the paternity, at a time when parents (confirmed mother and alleged father) are already unavailable for analysis. In this case, the autosomal genetic analysis may provide insufficient statistical robustness and the analysis of sex-related markers may be needed—see 3.b. Even considering that type of data, the genetic analyses may not provide sufficient information to satisfactorily discern between full- and half-sibship, at least considering the standard number of markers used in forensic casuistic.

3.b. Are John and Bill half-brothers?

From the point of view of diploid genetic transmission, paternal and maternal half-siblings are equally related, the individuals sharing with the same probability parental genetic information (possessing one pair of alleles with common ancestry, as parent-child), or not (possessing no alleles with common ancestry, as unrelated individuals). This high chance (50%) of not sharing any transmitted genetic information per diploid marker implies that such markers may provide weak statistical power to discriminate from the alternative hypothesis of being unrelated. Sex-linked markers may in this case be crucial depending on the sex of the involved individuals. In the case of half-brothers, as Bill and John, the analysis of Y chromosomal markers is useless if the questioned half-sibship is maternal (under both hypotheses, they do not share Y chromosome genetic information, as they have different fathers), contrary to X chromosomal ones, for which the probability of sharing the maternal genetic information is 50%. In both cases, either paternal or maternal half-sibship, lineage markers (Y chromosome and mtDNA in the first and second case, respectively) are powerful in providing evidence against the claimed kinship (or in favor of the alternative hypothesis of unrelatedness) when their genetic profiles do not match.

When the individuals analyzed are from opposite sexes, X chromosome markers may be used in the case of maternal half-sibship, since the probability of genetic sharing between half brother and sister is expected to be 50%.

In half-sibship problems, the use of X chromosome markers is particularly interesting in the case in which female individuals are analyzed, especially when the paternal kinship is disputed. Under this hypothesis, females share the entire X chromosomal paternal information unless mutation(s) occur, so, even using a modest number of markers it is likely to obtain very powerful statistical results. Indeed, the expected power in a paternal half-sister case (with 'unrelated' as the alternative hypothesis) when using X chromosomal markers is similar to the one obtained when using autosomal markers in a standard paternity duo test (again with 'unrelated' as the alternative hypothesis). However, in the case of maternal half-sisters, the power obtained with X chromosomal markers is comparable to the one obtained for autosomes and complementing these results may still be insufficient to obtain a statistically robust analysis. As a complimentary approach, maternally transmitted mtDNA may be analyzed, which can provide strong evidence, favoring the absence of the maternal relatedness, in case the profiles of the disputed maternal half-sisters do not match (see also Q&A 5 and 6).

4. Male lineage assignment: *Do John and Bill belong to the same paternal lineage?*

The question of belonging to a male lineage is not usually formulated in forensics as such by the requesting parties but is commonly translated into these terms in the course of many kinship investigations, namely as an ancillary tool, or to rule out alternative kinships, which are hard to distinguish using classical (diploid) genetic markers (BOXes 5 and 6). It can also happen that the evidence just provides reliable information on male limited, paternally transmitted (Y-chromosomal) genetic markers. These markers, due their distinctive transmission mode (BOX 6), while defining male lineages, do not allow individual identification. They can however be used in the establishment of genealogies, either for recreational purposes or as ancillary evidence in national citizenship claims.

Briefly, these markers are transmitted *en bloc* through the Y chromosome from fathers to sons—and to sons only (BOXes 5 and 6), so that all patrilineage related males share the same genetic profile (↑Glossary) unless mutations (↑Glossary) occur. Then, the specific Y chromosomal information of any male individual is the same as his father, paternal grandfather, paternal great grandfather, and so on, copy errors excepted. Consequently, Y chromosome specific markers are of utmost interest in anthropology as their tracking allows the determination of the males' migration routes. Unsurprisingly, there are currently many companies that provide male customers with an estimation of their bio-geographic ancestry by the analysis of this type of markers. Note that, from the Y chromosome specific marker's point of view, individuals with a close kinship, such as two maternal half-brothers, may be unrelated, and that kinship between individuals of different sex is always nil (BOXes 6 and 7).

In forensics, the male specific part of the Y chromosome is useful in a broad range of problems, specifically when autosomal markers (↑Glossary) provide little or no information at all. A common forensically relevant motivation for the analysis of these male lineage markers is that most sexually related crimes are committed by males on female victims. In theses cases, the specific recovery of genetic material from the male perpetrator, from a mixture in which female genetic

33

material is vastly predominant, is easier for Y chromosome markers. Albeit not allowing individual identification, these markers are crucial for: *(i)* excluding male suspects from their involvement in a crime, *(ii)* detecting multiple male contributors in a trace, *(iii)* identifying the paternal lineage of male perpetrators, or *(iv)* providing investigative leads of the paternal bio-geographic ancestry of unknown male perpetrators. The weighing of the hypothesis of two males having the same paternal lineage may arise in paternity disputes of male offspring (or other paternal kinships), including historical cases, as well as in identification cases in the scope of missing persons or mass disaster victims.

For the development of this chapter, we have chosen just one illustrative example that can be exploited in two settings: the first one is quite common in genealogical investigations, and the second in criminalistics.

Considering the weighing of the evidence, this peculiar, uniparental, mode of transmission, in contrast with biparentally transmitted markers, prevents the calculation of expected frequencies for genetic profiles. In fact, the genetic profile for these male exclusive markers behaves as a single, albeit complex and highly informative marker. Consequently, the quantification of its genetic evidence is purely empirical and extremely sensitive to questions of population sampling (BOX 9); the statistical confidence regarding the results relying on the quality of the existing population frequency data (BOX 15).

It should now be clear that the mode of transmission of the lineage markers pose serious questions to the combination of information obtained with other genetic data resulting from biparental markers. Indeed, while the latter is suitable to the formulation of hypotheses through individual identification, the Y chromosome is just able to identify a lineage, which is, by definition, a large set of individuals. The controversies regarding the ways of joining both types of information are presented in BOX 16.

4.a. Do John and Bill share the same male lineage?

Here, we suppose that the question is if the two individuals John and Bill belong to the same male lineage. We assume that we can type, or have access to, the Y chromosome genetic profiles from both males *and that they are identical* (we will analyze later the alternative outcome). If we were to proceed similarly to previous cases (Q&A 1, 2, and 3), the next step would involve the calculation of a likelihood ratio in which the numerator will be (**H1**) the frequency of John and Bill's genetic profile assuming they belong to the same paternal lineage. However, in contrast to the situations examined up to now, this frequency is directly estimated from repositories of data on the distribution of profiles observed in the population to which John and Bill belong (for simplicity we assume their geographical ancestry is known and the same) *and not an expected frequency*. The result of this data repository querying (BOX 15) will provide a result symbolized as $P(R|H1)$, which is simply *the frequency of the profile and of the lineage it defines* in the population at stake: number of occurrences of the profile in the repository/total number of repository samples.

As we will detail below, two individuals may indeed belong to the same lineage but display different profiles due to mutation (↑Glossary), which means that a formally correct calculation should include this possibility. Nevertheless, when profiles are coincident, the easiest way to convey the probatory value of the evidence consists in just reporting how frequent the profile is.

A possible reporting formulation would be:

Bill and John share the same genetic profile, consistent with belonging to the same paternal lineage, and the frequency of that profile, estimated by random sampling of size N of the population, is f.

Depending on the population and the number of markers typed to construct the profile, quite often the profile of the analyzed males is not reported or was found just once. If this occurs, a minimal frequency estimation: $f = 1/N$, is attributed to that genetic profile. This is due to the high level of polymorphism of the analyzed markers, which lead to a tremendous number of combinatorial possibilities for the genetic profiles of the individuals. The number of markers included in commercial kits has increased, currently ranging from 8 to 27 markers. Even considering the smallest number of markers (8), if we consider 10 possibilities for each one, this results in 10^8 possible genetic profiles, which were impossible to observe in the (much smaller) number of analyzed individuals.

Although surprising at first sight, is easy to understand that two individuals who indeed belong to the same male lineage may show different profiles due to the possible occurrence of mutations. Among others, the probability of observing mutations depends on the number and type of genetic markers included in the profile, and on the number of generations separating the two individuals. Indeed, for any type of genetic marker, the greater the numbers of these two (number of analyzed markers and generations separating the individuals), the smaller the chance to obtain exactly the same profile in a pair of individuals. For example, it is more likely to detect a mutation in a pair of paternal brothers (two genetic transmissions) than in a father-son duo (just one genetic transmission). Similarly, it is more likely to observe a mutation in a father-son duo if 27 markers, instead of 8, are analyzed. Reporting such a result of no coincidence is thus much more complex. Now we cannot avoid that the observation may have two explanations:

(a) Bill and John belong to the same paternal lineage (i.e., they have a recent common paternal ancestor, and the differences are attributed to mutations), or

(b) Bill and John do not belong to the same paternal lineage (i.e., they do not share a recent common paternal ancestor).

In other words, if we go back enough in time, *all extant lineages coalesce into a single ancestral one*, which explains why this formulation only makes sense under the hypothesis of the individuals being, or not, close paternal relatives, that is, sharing, or not, a *recent* common paternal ancestor. To calculate the expected frequencies of the observed profiles under the two alternative explanations, the knowledge of the number of generations separating Bill and John from the questioned common ancestor is therefore required, allowing the inclusion of the probability of the occurrence of mutations. For example, if Bill and John have supposedly the same father, for each marker there are only two opportunities for the occurrence of mutations, while if the common male ancestor is a grandfather, this number rises to four (the number of paternal transmissions). This means that the open question, "Do Bill and Joe belong to the same lineage?" is too vague and a specific kinship must be assumed and two alternative kinship hypotheses (H1, main, and H2, alternative) must be considered. H1 would then be, for example, "Bill and John are paternal brothers", and H2 "Bill and John are not paternally related". In this case, note that the main and alternative hypotheses are not mutually exclusive and exhaustive: that is, Bill and John could be paternally related more remotely (as, for instance, cousins). In consequence, *this formulation is only acceptable if brotherhood is the only possible kinship between Bill and John*. Again, since all of us, Bill and John included, share a distant common ancestor, stating that no other kinship exists means *close* kinship, which in practical terms means that the sum of the number of generations separating Bill and John from the common ancestor is greater than six (common ancestor great-grandfather). The expected frequency of the observations under the first hypothesis $P(R \mid H1)$ would then be calculated assuming the specific kinship and the occurrence of mutation, and the one under the alternative $P(R \mid H2)$ as the probability of finding the profiles at random in the population. A likelihood ratio, LR, could then be computed, and a possible reporting formulation would be:

> *The observed results are LR times more likely assuming that Bill and John are paternal brothers than considering them as unrelated.*

If the LR assumes a value below 1, it means that the observations are more likely if the individuals are not closely paternally related.

Conversely—and more disturbingly, two individuals belonging to different lineages may show the same genetic profile. The probability of this occurrence decreases with the increase of the analyzed markers, also depending on the mutation rates of the markers. Indeed, if it is true that mutation can cause two paternally related males to exhibit different genetic information, it is also true that two paternally unrelated individuals, with different genetic ancestors, may exhibit the same genetic state due to convergent mutations.

These facts seriously complicate the interpretation of the comparisons between profiles and consequently their forensic evaluation. The conclusion is that the correct forensic evaluation of Y-chromosome profiles requires not only prohibitively extensive databases, but also accurate estimates of *mutation rates*. The latter still more difficult to obtain as they require not random simple populational samples, but pairs of guaranteed paternally related individuals (usually father/son pairs).

4.b. Do the suspect and the crime scene sample share the same paternal lineage?

Let us now consider that a perfect match is obtained between the Y chromosome profiles from a crime scene sample and one from a suspect (or from an individual profile stored in a human forensic DNA database). Now we can follow the standard procedure of establishing a likelihood ratio, but under a different type of hypothesis. For the numerator H1, the formulation could be: "The crime scene sample was left by the suspect or by some close paternal relative of his", while the alternative H2 would be: "The crime scene sample was left by a random male, not closely related paternally to the suspect". P(R|H1) corresponds then to the frequency F of the profile in the population (f), and P(R|H2) to the probability of finding two individuals belonging to the same lineage ($F \times F$). The ratio

$$LR = P(R|H1)/P(R|H2),$$

will then take the value of

$$1/F$$

and the result could be verbally translated into:

The genetic observations are LR times more probable assuming that the crime scene sample was left by the donor of the reference sample, or by some close paternal relative of his, than assuming it was left by a paternally unrelated individual.

Note that this value can only be used to confirm the suspicion, provided the other possible contributors from the same lineage are ruled out by the results of an investigation of non-genetic evidence.

FURTHER INFO

Willuweit, S. and Roewer, L. (2007, Jun). International Forensic Y Chromosome User Group. Y chromosome haplotype reference database (YHRD): Update. Forensic Sci. Int. Genet., 1(2): 83–7. doi: 10.1016/j.fsigen.2007.01.017.

Willuweit, S. and Roewer, L. (2015). The new Y Chromosome haplotype reference database. Forensic Science International Genetics, 15: 43–48. https://doi.org/10.1016/j.fsigen.2014.11.024.

5. Female lineage assignment: *Do John and Anna belong to the same maternal lineage?*

As with what happens to the paternal counterpart (II.4), the question of individuals belonging to the same maternal lineage is very infrequently formulated by the requesting parties. It is however commonly translated in the wording used in the title of this section in many FG investigations, in most of the cases as an auxiliary tool to identification or kinship establishment. For example, two adopted children, now adults, may be interested in weighing the possibility of being maternally related.

If Y chromosomal markers are useful to identify paternal lineages, being transmitted *en block* from fathers to sons, markers transmitted via mitochondrial DNA (mtDNA; ↑Glossary; BOXes 1, 5, and 6) may be used to disclose maternal lineages since they are transmitted from mothers to both daughters and sons (but *males do not transmit it*). Thus, a mother shares the same mtDNA profile with all her offspring, unless mutations (↑Glossary) occur. This implies that somewhat distant relatives may share the same mtDNA profile, as is the case, for example, of two female second cousins, daughters of a pair of (female) first cousins, daughters of a pair of full sisters (they share the mtDNA of the common great-grandmother, unless mutations occur). Conversely, from the mtDNA point of view, closely related individuals may equate to being unrelated, as is the case of fathers concerning both daughters and sons (BOXes 6 and 7).

Indeed, as for the Y chromosome, it may be useful to study mtDNA because it utilizes genetic markers with a particular mode of transmission (BOXes 5 and 6), and does not allow individual identification. The main difference from Y-chromosome transmission in this quasi symmetry resides in it being possible to compare persons of both sexes, while in exclusively male-mediated transmission, only males are usefully analyzable.

Again, as for the Y chromosome, this mode of inheritance does not allow the calculation of expected frequencies for genetic profiles, and these maternally transmitted markers behave as a single one, being inherited as a whole. In consequence, the quantification of the genetic evidence from mtDNA is purely empirical and extremely sensitive to questions of population structure (although a little less than the male counterpart) and the statistical confidence in the results depends on the quality of the existing databases, being much more sensitive to such biases than biparentally transmitted markers (BOXes 5, 9, and 15). This occurs because the individual genetic profiles must be analyzed as a whole, which requires much greater population databases than when markers (likely belonging to different chromosomes) are independently analyzed from each other, which is generally the case for the diploid markers standardly used in identification and kinship problems. Identical to the Y chromosome, these characteristics pose serious questions to the combination of information obtained from mtDNA with other genetic data types (see BOX 16).

There is however a forensically more relevant motivation for mtDNA analysis: It is reliably retrievable from old, degraded, and/or minute samples for which all other types of markers fail to produce results using validated protocols. For example, mtDNA may be particularly useful in mass disaster victims' identification, where genetic information may be recovered from hair, bones, or teeth that typically contain low concentrations of (degraded) DNA, making them unsuitable for nuclear DNA examinations.

In a manner symmetrical to paternal lineage markers, applications of mtDNA include the establishment of the maternal lineage which may support the ruling out of maternal kinships or sample contributions. There is however a major difference between the two types of markers, concerning both the mode of transmission and technical difficulties.

Indeed, while all other types of genetic markers are present in a fixed number of copies per cell (zero, one, or two), mtDNA occurs in a high and *variable* number of copies (BOX 1). Furthermore, mutations (errors in DNA duplication, ↑Glossary) are highly frequent. Consequently, it is much more likely to find, in the same individual, different types of mtDNA than for any other type of marker, and a specific word was coined for the phenomenon: *heteroplasmy* (↑Glossary, BOX 11). This difficulty is however not insurmountable as, except in rare cases, its presence does not preclude a safe assignment of the transmitted mtDNA to a maternal lineage.

Bearing this caution in mind, we will not repeat what was explained for paternal lineages assignment (Q&A 4), kindly asking the reader to replace 'paternal' with 'maternal' and 'Y chromosome' with 'mtDNA'.

FURTHER INFO

Connell, J.R., Benton, M.C., Lea, R.A., Sutherland, H.G., Haupt, L.M. and Wright, K.M. (2022). Evaluating the suitability of current mitochondrial DNA interpretation guidelines for multigenerational whole mitochondrial genome comparisons. J. Forensic Sci., 00: 1– 10. https://doi.org/10.1111/1556-4029.15097.

McElhoe, J.A., Wilton, P.R., Parson, W. and Holland, M.M. (2022, May). Exploring statistical weight estimates for mitochondrial DNA matches involving heteroplasmy. Int. J. Legal Med., 136(3): 671–685. doi: 10.1007/s00414-022-02774-5.

Parson, W. and Dür, A. (2007, Jun). EMPOP--a forensic mtDNA database. Forensic Sci. Int. Genet., 1(2): 88–92. doi: 10.1016/j.fsigen.2007.01.018.

6. Non-human identification: *Is this item from an individual non-human living being?*

In FG, the identification of any kind of living being would be expected to be formally identical to the methodology used for humans, as discussed in II.1. There are, however, some relevant differences and exceptions which have to do with the variety of reproductive modes we can find across the tree of life.

Therefore, we must examine the known modes of biological reproduction and associated modes of transmission (BOXes 1, 2, and 5), in order to be able to decide if, when, how, and which approaches developed for humans can be applied to other species and organisms.

Table II.6.1 summarizes what is the current knowledge on this matter, depicting only the most widespread reproduction modes; many others are indeed known (see BOX 1 for the basic concepts, biological mechanisms and definitions of the terms employed; for an overview on the diversity of the life and the special case of viruses, see BOX 18). The purpose of presenting this here is simply to allow a glimpse on their variety and complexity.

Table 6.1. Known reproductive and genetic transmission modes found in the current Earth biosphere. Details and limitations are discussed at BOX 18.

Reproduction mode	Transmission modes	Organisms	Comments
ASEXUAL	Uniparental	Bacteria Plants Animals Fungi	Many prokaryotes are capable of parasexuality. Many animals, fungi and plants reproduce sexually and/or asexually.
SEXUAL	Uniparental	Plants Animals Fungi	Most eukaryotes are symbionts in which the organelles (mitochondria, plastids) reminiscent of the once free-living prokaryote have, with few known exceptions, uniparental transmission.
	Biparental homogametic	Plants Animals Fungi	The most employed and preferred transmission mode in standard forensic genetics.
	Biparental heterogametic	Animals	The X chromosome markers found in mammals.

Keeping this variety in mind, it is easy to understand that any FG application to an organism requires a previous investigation of its biology. This has been extensively performed for *Homo sapiens*, but that knowledge is only available for a handful of other species—mainly those of economic interest or model organisms used in biological/ biomedical scientific research, data being especially meager on wildlife. In fact, there are many groups of organisms for which the concept of individual identification is genetically meaningless. It suffices to recall that a substantial part of the biosphere is capable of clonal (↑Glossary) reproduction and in many cases, they are exclusively resorting to it to propagate. The most common example is the one found in many plants, in which a part of it can (grafted into another plant or just put in the soil) generate a new, complete, and independent individual. *The individuals resulting from this cloning process are therefore genetically identical and consequently, indistinguishable.*

This warning made another cautionary note essential: The use of FG for identification purposes also requires that the population genetics studies be performed on the targeted species and that typing methods and protocols were validated. Again, we are extremely far from reaching this state, apart from a few domesticates.

Fortunately, the members of domesticated species—including pets or plants—are the organisms most used as silent witnesses, providing precious associative evidence in criminal investigations. For example, in a case where cat hairs are found on the clothes of a victim, experts may want to genetically test if they were shed by the suspect's pet. Domesticates are also involved in most of the cases requiring the identification of the animal responsible for property damage, body offenses (or even death), as well as in a plethora of other issues of forensic relevance, such as doping of sports animals or fraud in the pedigree of highly priced pets. It must be said, however, that the analysis of non-human genetic data presents specific problems for FG, due to the profound impact of the process of domestication on their genetic diversity. Indeed, their controlled reproduction, selection, and inbreeding prevent a straightforward extension of the simple models used in humans for the calculation of expected frequencies of genetic profiles.

Having these limitations in mind, we will illustrate the case where the genetic evidence provided by a sufficiently studied species is used to indirectly contribute to identifying a human perpetrator, or in which a specific animal needs to be identified to confirm if it was responsible for an attack or property damage.

In both situations, the question addressable by FG is formally identical to those we have already analyzed for human identification (cf. II.1. a. *Identification: comparison of genetic profiles between trace and suspect*), and can be stated as:

Is the questioned sample from a determined organism?

As for humans, we will assume that the material evidence to be genetically analyzed is genuine, uncontaminated, and presented in sufficient amount and good preservation conditions. Identically, it is supposed that the genetic profile of the individual organism putatively involved is known or obtainable during the investigation. Likewise, we assume that the genetic profiles are defined by biparentally transmitted (BOX 5) genetic markers (BOX 3), as in the human case.

It will then be possible to compare the genetic profile found in the vestige with the one from the questioned individual organism (both analyzed during the case or using a previously typed profile of the individual organism).

The result of the comparison may be that the two profiles are identical. If this is the case, it will be reported in the form of a ratio, in which the numerator is the expected frequency of the profile in the relevant population, or the probability of finding, at random, this genetic profile (↑Glossary), under the hypothesis **H1**: They are from the same individual organism, which is symbolized as: P(O|H1) (read as: the probability of the observation given, or assuming, H1). The denominator is the expected frequency of the same profile in a random pair of individuals in the relevant population, assuming therefore the alternative hypothesis, **H2**: the questioned organism and the vestige donor are distinct individuals randomly sampled in the relevant population, and accordingly symbolized as P(O|H2).

Then, the reported result, usually called **likelihood ratio**, will be

$$LR = P(O|H1)/P(O|H2)$$

which can be phrased as: The genetic observations are LR times more probable assuming the sample is from the questioned individual organism, than assuming it came from another, genetically unrelated individual (BOX 14).

LR is *not* a probability, although it can be converted into it, using the Bayes' theorem (BOX 14). This conversion is however complex, involving more assumptions and the unnecessary risk of conflicting with the independence of the expert, by involving the formulation of prior probabilities, as happens when dealing with humans.

Note that the calculation of the expected frequencies above requires previous genetic information on the relevant population, that is, reliable estimates of the parameters involved (BOX 9). This requirement may be much more difficult to satisfy than for humans, due to the lack of studies on the population genetics of the species. More importantly, population structure, a minor problem in humans, due to the relatively low interpopulation differences in the frequencies of the genetic markers used, is serious in most wild and domesticated animals and plants, in which genetic races do often exist. In other words, while the expectation of the rarity of an individual genetic profile in humans is slightly affected by the inadequate use of a database (e.g., African instead of Eurasian), this is not so for other species, as it is especially visible in the case of domesticates, such as dogs. Indeed, strict mating rules were maintained over centuries to select the desired dog breeds, developed to obtain specimens with specific characteristics. The genetic characteristics of two dogs from different breeds are then expected to differ more greatly than a pair of humans from different continents. When the result of the comparison is that the two profiles are not identical, it would seem at first sight that a categorical conclusion is possible: that the two profiles have certainly different donors (BOX 17). As for humans (II.1), the situation is not so simple, as it has been observed that distinct parts of one individual organism can exhibit different genetic profiles, due to somatic mutation (↑Glossary), leading to mosaicism, (↑Glossary), or to chimerism (↑Glossary).

The solution to this problem is also more difficult than in humans due to poorer knowledge and informative power of the fewer validated genetic markers available.

Finally, and again as for humans, if mosaicism is admitted as an explanation for the (few) differences between the profiles, the numerator of the ratio above must be generalized to incorporate this possibility, that is, the occurrence of mutation(s).

MORE INFO

Amorim, A. and Budowle, B. (2016). Handbook of Forensic Genetics: Biodiversity and Heredity in Civil and Criminal Investigation. World Scientific, New Jersey.

Arenas, M., Pereira, F., Oliveira, M., Pinto, N., Lopes, A.M., Gomes, V., Carracedo, A. and Amorim, A. (2017). Forensic Genetics and Genomics: Much More than just a Human Affair. PLoS Genet., 13(9): e1006960.

7. Taxonomic identification: *Is this item from a given species?*

Classification of living organisms is still a matter of debate among specialists, despite the revolutionary impact of genetics on the understanding of biological evolution (BOX 18). The controversies still rage, starting at the definition of the conceptually most basic building block—what is a species? The most accepted definition, "Species are groups of interbreeding natural populations that are reproductively isolated from other such groups," only applies to a very small fraction of life forms, those with obligatory sexual reproduction. Note that this definition (commonly named as the biological definition of species) does not consider visible characteristics, but simply their genetic transmission: "the degree of morphological difference is not appropriate for species definition" [MAYR 1996].

But more fundamentally, even when considering just this subset of sexually reproducing organisms, taxonomists diverge on the evolutionarily dynamic nature of a species, some considering it as a conceptual freezing of a diversity continuum without biological meaning. If we were to follow this view on the distribution of biological diversity, FG would have very little, if anything, to do— species assignment would be impossible or arbitrary, since there would be no way to define distinctive genetic profiles. The truth is however that the observed distribution of genetic diversity is discrete, at least for the vast majority of sexually reproducing organisms. It would therefore seem possible—leastwise for this share of the living world, to design genetic tests able to answer the question of specific assignment. This conclusion is based on the premise that the definition and naming of a species is consensual among taxonomists, following unambiguous criteria. This is sadly not the case: most classifications were and are still made on the base of morphological criteria that have little correlation with the genetic definition of species. Some specialists consider that "the classification of complex organisms is in chaos" and even "if species delineations are at least partly arbitrary, deliberations must draw on expertise beyond taxonomy, morphology, systematics and *genetics* [our italics]," so that "any definition can withstand legal challenge" [GARNETT and CHRISTIDIS 2017].

This somewhat chaotic situation is unfortunately so common that it applies to groups including domesticates and protected wild species (such as canids, or pigs/boars), transforming the task of FG in helping law enforcement extremely hard to accomplish.

An extra difficulty arises from the fact that many publicly available DNA databases containing taxonomically relevant information may not be properly curated, containing errors which will hamper their forensic use. Regardless of these limitations, those resources allow the comparison between the genetic profile of an unidentified sample and those stored in the database associated with a certain species.

The cooperative efforts into constructing genetic databases for the world species have been centered on uniparentally transmitted markers. The most relevant is the Consortium for the Barcode of Life [https://ibol.org/about/dna-barcoding/], which includes biparental markers only for plants and fungi. The consequence of the limited availability of animal data to mtDNA (which is almost universally maternally transmitted) is that the corresponding genetic tests fail to identify hybrids. For instance, the species assignment of a sample obtained from a mule (sterile offspring of a male donkey and a female horse) would classify it as horse (*Equus caballus*), while a hinny (the offspring of the symmetrical crossing between a male horse and a female donkey) would be assigned to *Equus asinus*, the donkey.

The data availability, along with mtDNA being more abundant and easier to be reliably typed in critical samples, explain why almost all FG developments aimed at species identification use it, despite its limitations and pitfalls.

We will therefore limit our analysis to a couple of fictitious examples using the most popular approaches (the abovementioned DNA Barcode approach and the SpInDel method) to species assignment, employing uniparentally transmitted markers, mitochondrial (in the case of animals) or plastid (plants) DNA, and evidencing their pros, cons and applicability.

For that we will suppose that the species of origin of a morphologically uninformative sample is questioned. This is often the case for many real-life situations, such as the confiscation, at borders, of skins, eggs, powders, etc., which provide scarce or no relevant information from morphological examination, due to the suspicion of their being from a protected species.

In many of those cases, the suspicion on the seized material provenance is grounded on vague evidence, such as the behavior of the carrier and officers do not have any clue about the putative protected species (one or various) nor of broader taxonomic group(s). In such a situation, the contribution of FG is much more difficult than if the suspicion is narrowed down to a single (or a limited number of) species. We will explain this with the simplest type of case, using animal examples, which are, by far the commonest in forensic focus:

7.a Does this item contain material from the protected species X?

There is a suspicion that some seized item contains material from the protected animal species X; for example, powder suspected to contain a rhinoceros's horn. So, the responsibility placed on FG is to help to prove it. Since a single species is targeted, the current strategy is to type the sample aiming at the genetic marker available in the DNA Barcode database (preferably) or other repositories (as GenBank). There exist specific, standardized protocols for that purpose and if the sample indeed contains material from the questioned species, mtDNA information (in the form of a sequence) is obtained and compared with the reference at the database (via the BOLD platform itself, which provides the informatic tool publicly). We will non-exhaustively review the possible outcomes of this analysis:

Outcome 1: There is a good chance that, even after repeated essays, no sequence (or any reliable genetic information) is obtained from the biological sample under investigation, and the resulting report will sadly conclude something like:

> *Using the standard protocols, which are virtually universal in the detection of animal DNA, and namely from the suspected species X, it was impossible to obtain any reliable information.*

This (lack of) result may be due to either absence of DNA or to its presence in so small an amount and/or so degraded as to reach the detection threshold (and, for some popular typing techniques, the presence of chemical inhibitors, BOX 13).

Outcome 2: In case of full identity with (and only with) the target species, a typical expert report will be:

The item contains genetic material whose sequence is identical to one referenced as corresponding to species X in the BOLD database, and the nearest match with a different species showed low (e.g., 60%) similarity.

It seems that this conclusion is clear and unambiguous: the analyzed sequence is exactly the same as the one corresponding to a single species and all sequences present in the queried database are very different, as the nearest most similar sequences show differences in a large proportion of positions compared (possible pitfalls will be discussed in the end of the section, along with sometimes hidden assumptions).

Outcome 3: But it may also happen that the identity is not total and then the report would conclude something as:

The item contains genetic material whose sequence is (e.g.) 98.0% identical to one referenced as corresponding to the species X in the BOLD database, and the nearest match with a different species showed low (e.g., 60%) similarity.

Now the conclusion is less assertive, but nonetheless useful if not enabling a safe decision.

Outcome 4: It may as well happen that the database search retrieves a not so clear-cut picture, as when two (or more) species are found with highly similar, but non-identical profile to the one found in the sample. In such a case, the report would state:

The item contains genetic material whose sequence is (e.g.) 95% identical to sequences referenced as corresponding to species X and Y in the BOLD database, and the nearest match with a different species showed low (e.g., 60%) similarity.

Now the usefulness of the analysis is obviously lower since the identity is imperfect and the assignment ambiguous for two species, a result particularly undesirable if species Y is not under protection. Moreover, it may also be that (a) the true donor species is not in the database, or (b) X and Y are genetically very diverse and/or they are not true species, that is, they should be classified as a single taxonomic unit (according to the genetic definition of a species mentioned above).

Outcome 5: Another possible outcome: the material reveals a sequence quite different from the queried species, X, but identical (or showing a very high similarity) to a different one, Z, a result that could be reported as:

> *The item contains genetic material whose sequence shows very limited (e.g., 60%) similarity to sequence(s) referenced as corresponding to species X in the BOLD database and is 100% identical to the one referenced as corresponding to species Z in the same database.*

Here the result, although negative to the prosecution, is again clear-cut in pointing out as donor of a different species (which may or may not be under protection).

Outcome 6: There remains (besides the total incapacity of obtaining a clear profile, or the ambiguity in some positions at the sequence, to be discussed below) the situation of finding a sequence without any significant identity proportion in the entire database, which could be reported as:

> *The item contains genetic material whose sequence shows no significant similarity to sequence(s) referenced as corresponding to species X, as well as to any sequence stored in the BOLD database.*

Now we have a truly negative result, since not only species X seems ruled out, but also no alternative assignment is suggested. We may say that such a result is highly unlikely, despite the relative low coverage of the wild fauna of some geographic areas. Indeed, the current state of BOLD database is believed to embrace the major animal groups, and so some more or less similar sequence belonging to an evolutionary relative of the donor of the retrieved sequence is expected to have been deposited. Admittedly, this is less true for small animals (such as nematodes and other worms), neglected in conservation policies and for remote ecological niches (not only on land, but in also in marine environments, and particularly so at deep sea). If it is difficult to attribute the strange outcome to some technical or human error, the origin of a sequence with these characteristics may deserve a dedicated investigation, as it may reveal an unknown ramification of the animal branch in the tree of life.

In the fictitious cases described above, we have assumed the absence of *(i)* human or technical errors, *(ii)* chain-of-custody breaches, *(iii)* contamination, and *(iv)* ambiguities in the detected sequence. It was also assumed that no other species possess the same sequence as the queried one, and that no multiple animal sources contributed to the item with unbalanced quantities. Despite sometimes not explicitly stated, all these assumptions are also established in real forensic cases.

7.b. *A cautionary note on the common hidden assumptions and pitfalls*

We have assumed in all fictitious cases, as it happens in real life, sometimes not explicitly stated, the absence of:

- human or technical errors,
- chain-of-custody breaches,
- contamination,
- ambiguities in the detected sequence,
- conflicting or inconsistent taxonomy (internal to the database or with the queried species),
- an unknown species other than the queried one possessing the same sequence,
- multiple animal sources of the item contributing with unbalanced quantities.

Some of these assumptions are frequently not met, thus compromising the validity of the results. In this regard, it must be said that FG practices tend to be less stringent when dealing with non-human materials, either because the forensic lab in charge is not used to non-human materials and associated problems and/or, conversely, because the analysis is conducted in a laboratory not familiar with forensic framework.

FURTHER INFO

Alves, C., Pereira, R., Prieto, L., Aler, M., Amaral, C.R.L., Arévalo, C., Berardi, G., Di Rocco, F., Caputo, M., Carmona, C.H., Catelli, L., Costa, H.A., Coufalova, P., Furfuro, S., García, Ó., Gaviria, A., Goios, A., Gómez, J.J.B., Hernández, A., Hernández, E.D.C.B., Miranda, L., Parra, D., Pedrosa, S., Porto, M.J.A., Rebelo,

M.L., Spirito, M., Torres, M.D.C.V., Amorim, A. and Pereira, F. (2017). Species identification in forensic samples using the SPInDel approach: A GHEP-ISFG inter-laboratory collaborative exercise. Forensic Sci. Int. Genet., 28: 219–224. doi: 10.1016/j.fsigen.2017.03.003.

Arenas, M., Pereira, F., Oliveira, M., Pinto, N., Lopes, A.M., Gomes, V., Carracedo, A. and Amorim, A. (2017). Forensic genetics and genomics: Much more than just a human affair. PLoS Genet., 13(9): e1006960. doi: 10.1371/journal.pgen.1006960.

Garnett, S.T. and Christidis, L. (2017). Taxonomy anarchy hampers conservation. Nature, 546(7656): 25–27. doi: 10.1038/546025a.

Linacre, A. (2021). Animal forensic genetics. Genes (Basel)., 12(4): 515. doi: 10.3390/genes12040515.

Linacre, A., Gusmão, L., Hecht, W., Hellmann, A., Mayr, W., Parson, W., Prinz, M., Schneider, P. and Morling, N. (2011). ISFG: Recommendations regarding the use of non-human (animal) DNA in forensic genetic investigations. Forensic Sci. Int. Genet., 5: 501–505.

Mayr, E. (1996). What Is a Species, and What Is Not? Philosophy of Science, 63(2): 262–277. http://www.jstor.org/stable/188473.

Mukherjee, S., Huntemann, M., Ivanova, N. et al. (2015). Large-scale contamination of microbial isolate genomes by Illumina PhiX control. Stand in Genomic Sci. 10: 18. https://doi.org/10.1186/1944-3277-10-18.

8. Does the food label correctly describes the contents?

This section supposes the readers' knowledge of the contents of the previous one, which summarizes the specific difficulties of FG when dealing with non-human materials. Here we will extend the analysis to the contribution of FG to a growing demand of assessment and control of food quality and safety.

Corresponding to a part of this complex demand, FG can provide an answer to the questions of authenticity and labeling conformity of products of biological origin, and only those (detection of chemical, abiological adulteration is out of FG scope of action). The currently hot topic of the presence of material from genetically modified organisms (GMOs ↑Glossary, BOX 19), will be treated separately due to its specificity (II.9 Is the product of a genetically modified organism present in the item?)

These two aspects materialize into two types of questions: (*i*) Does the product contain the biological material from the organism(s) described in the label? and, (*ii*) does the product contain biological material from the organism(s) not mentioned in the label (and supposed to be absent)?

Some cautionary notes are, however, necessary before proceeding. Firstly, it must be clear that in many cases (as after intensive food processing), it may happen that the chemical modification of the biological material may hamper its detection by current FG-validated methods. Secondly, any analytical technique has its own detection threshold level, which means that if the quantity of the targeted contribution is too low, it may well go unnoticed. The problem is aggravated in structured materials, for which the distribution of the components may be very heterogeneous; some parts of the item being enriched in some components and completely void of others. In contrast with most dairy products, for which this problem is usually unimportant, many common processed foods present it in high degree, such as sausages, hamburgers and so on. The issue is magnified if regulations quantitatively specify limits (maxima or minima) to the specific contributions—for example, when the product labelled as "wild pig sausage" is allowed to contain some specified proportion of meat or fat from other sources.

8.a. Does the product contain the biological material from the organism(s) described in the label?

In this case, the question is addressed just to the presence of material from a well defined and limited number of organisms and the FG contribution to answer it is straightforward.

It is assumed therefore that the contribution of other organisms, which may be present, even abundantly, is not questioned. Accordingly, to avoid misunderstandings, the question would be more precisely and unambiguously formulated as: *Are the products of the species listed in the labeled present in the item?* For example, was goat milk (much more expensive) used to produce a cheese in which label indicates its presence along with (cheaper) milk from other species?

That being the question, the problem is solved in the same manner as discussed in Chapter II. 7, in which we answered to: is this biological item from a given species? Here, the only difference consists in the number of organisms to be detected, while before a single source was considered. Consequently, we will not repeat the discussion on the limitations and pitfalls that may be involved, which are essentially the same.

8.b. Does the product contain biological material from the organism(s) not mentioned in the label (and supposed to be absent)?

This question is most of the time posed in the context of religious prohibitions or dietary restrictions. For the first, we can cite the Jewish and Islamic traditions, which forbid pork, and for the second, vegetarian limitations on products of animal origin.

Searching for the presence of a specific product origin, such as questioning if the item contains pork, is trivial and again refers us to the previously debated question (8.a.; see also Q&A 7) with the difference that the searched species of origin is not in the product label but is suspected to be included. Therefore, we will not repeat it here.

The problem is less tractable when the suspicion to be investigated is broad, including a sometimes enormously diverse range of organisms. If, for instance, we are searching for the presence of a product of animal origin, it is exceedingly difficult to design a test which will be able to detect specifical material with such a widely defined origin, excluding simultaneously all non-animal possible sources. Despite the incomplete coverage of genome sequencing across the tree of life, it is already quite clear that it is nearly impossible to achieve such a test, given the huge diversification observed among and across the traditional biological kingdoms, animals, plants and fungi (BOX 18).

Consequently, and being aware of the high risk of false positives as well as false negatives among the results of such an ambitious test, it is common to narrow the scope of the search to more manageable proportions. An example of such refocusing is the search of products promoted as vegetarian for the presence of material from a more reduced set of organisms, as land vertebrates (considered the possible producers of commonly called 'meat').

Even under this severely reduced range of possible donors (excluding therefore all fishes and shellfishes) what we already know from the genomes of a small number of land vertebrates has demonstrated the difficulty of designing a test able to reliably detect the presence of their products in an item.

An extra difficulty—and another source of misunderstanding—arises from the fact that most FG tests, if reliably assessing the type of organism, do not discriminate the type of product. That happens if the technique addresses the genetic origin (e.g., a land vertebrate), but not discriminate if the detected material is from milk, egg, or meat. That can be relevant for some dietary restriction rules, some of which tolerate dairy products, but not meat, for instance. Although some methods have been developed intending to resolve that distinction (as the detection of milk casein, or meat myosin), their use is not widespread, and should be always used in conjunction with DNA tests.

FURTHER INFO

Alves, C., Pereira, R., Prieto, L., Aler, M., Amaral, C.R.L., Arévalo, C., Berardi, G., Di Rocco, F., Caputo, M., Carmona, C.H., Catelli, L., Costa, H.A., Coufalova, P., Furfuro, S., García, Ó., Gaviria, A., Goios, A., Gómez, J.J.B., Hernández, A., Hernández, E.D.C.B., Miranda, L., Parra, D., Pedrosa, S., Porto, M.J.A., Rebelo, M.L., Spirito, M., Torres, M.D.C.V., Amorim, A. and Pereira, F. (2017). Species identification in forensic samples using the SPInDel approach: A GHEP-ISFG inter-laboratory collaborative exercise. Forensic Sci. Int. Genet., 28: 219–224. doi: 10.1016/j.fsigen.2017.03.003.

Gonçalves, J., Pereira, F., Amorim, A. and van Asch, B. (2012). New method for the simultaneous identification of cow, sheep, goat, and water buffalo in dairy products by analysis of short species-specific mitochondrial DNA targets. J. Agric. Food Chem., 60(42): 10480–5. doi: 10.1021/jf3029896.

9. Is the product of a genetically modified organism present in the item?

At first sight, it would seem that questioning the presence of a product from a genetically modified organism (GMO, ↑Glossary) would be frameable into previously analyzed problems, when addressing the detection of genetic material from specific organisms as constituents of a piece of evidence (II.7 and II.8).

This is however not the case, due to the ambiguity and diversity of GMOs legal definitions and many other factors (BOX 19).

Indeed, FG can only contribute an answer to the question if

(a) the biotechnological method used creates detectable, univocal, changes on the genetic material of the organism, and/or

(b) the genetic modification determines the synthesis of a detectable specific product, absent from the unmodified organism.

These conditions are not met when some of the recent techniques of genetic modifications are used (BOX 19) and therefore their detection is essentially impossible. But even when more classical processes are used, and detection is feasible, any analytical forensic approach (either addressing the process or the product of the genetic modification), requires the exact specification of the searched genetic modification.

An answerable problem through an FG approach would be, for instance, to know if an organism (or a derived foodstuff) is (or contains) genetically modified by a (either authorized or not) specific technique. A more concrete example would be:

Does this batch of frozen potato puree contain material from the GMO code X?

This question is now answered in the same way FG deals with known genetic markers (↑Glossary) and proceeds in an analogous way as described for food authenticity (Chapter II.8).

The problems and pitfalls are essentially the same, with the difference that what is now targeted for detection is, instead of species-specific genetic markers, the region of the genome altered by the X coded genetic alteration.

It must be stressed anyway that *the report, being negative, besides the limitations and pitfalls pointed out before for FG analysis in general (see BOX 13), does not allow to conclude that no (unauthorized) GMO product is present, but that just the specified one is absent.*

III
Questions without Answers
& Answers without Questions

Questions without Answers
& Answers without Questions

Since the introduction of DNA technologies and computational capabilities Forensic Genetics has gained an impetus that, based upon many spectacular achievements, has created the belief that this branch of auxiliary science of justice would be a universal problem solver, driving all other forensic sciences into obsolescence.

This belief, reinforced by abundantly publicized results in the media, creating unrealistic expectations on FG investigation techniques, is particularly dangerous, since it is widely shared among judicial actors, as jurors, judges, and lawyers. The importance of this overrated and misplaced understanding of FG was recognized by the researchers of the sociology of the administration of justice, who coined the expression "CSI effect" for the phenomenon, alluding to the title of a TV series especially responsible for it.

Misconceptions on FG possibilities and limitations exceed however this effect and, more seriously, they are also present among FG practitioners. FG experts sometimes overlook technical limitations (such as detection limits, or the possibility of artefactual or, in general terms, erroneous results, BOX 13), use incorrect formal and/or biostatistical approaches (BOX 14), or even over evaluate their own role in the legal proceedings, practicing decisional reporting styles and formats (BOX 17).

Aiming to minimize the impact of these misconceptions, it would be useful to identify the types of situations in which they are most likely to occur. We will try to do so by classifying them into two categories: (i) those arising from badly or ambiguously formulated questions or which, although sensible and well expressed, are out of FG reach, at least in the present state of the art, and *(ii)* the situations in which investigative activities autonomously create potential answers to unposed questions.

Questions without answers

As briefly discussed before at the Introduction, problems of communication are currently a major concern, not only on the side of the legal stakeholders, of understanding of the FG expert report, but also on the FG expert comprehension of the questions they asked to answer.

On the difficulties of correctly interpreting forensic genetic data by laypersons, the major obstacles have been identified, and corrective actions to improve the readability of FG reporting have been put forward, but for the most part are far from being consensual among experts and thus are not generally implemented.

But the main issue, as illustrated by the classical relevant question of criminalistics: *is X the author of the crime?* (II.1) is essentially out of FG capacity, by two main reasons: *(i)* FG does not provide individualization (Introduction/What is FG?) and *(ii)* is not entitled to assess the action or its criminal nature (Introduction/Levels and hierarchy of propositions). In other words, FG can contribute to answer the relevant question in just a very indirect and comparative way. This answer simply states (or should state, as is now quite generally recommended) that, *given the genetic profile from a piece of evidence allegedly associated with the crime*, the comparison of the probability (or expected frequencies) of the occurrence of that genetic profile in a single individual (the author and the suspect are the same person) with the probability of finding the same genetic profile in two individuals (author and suspect are not the same). If the results are reported in this manner (for details see II.1) it seems there is little room for misinterpretations, particularly if a frequency ratio formulation instead of conditional probabilities is adopted, but unfortunately this is not always the case.

Fallacious interpretations are troublingly common, most of them partaking the same basic error of mistaking the reported ratio as a probability, and/or misunderstanding conditional probabilities. The one known as the *transposed conditional fallacy*, wrongfully takes the result as the *probability of the hypothesis given the data*, instead of the *probability of the data given the hypothesis*. Whatever the kind of fallacy (including *prosecution and defense fallacies*) they highlight the danger of reporting FG results in a probability or probability-looking-like format. On the other hand, invoking Bayesian (posterior) probabilities, besides being frightening and incomprehensible to laypersons and judicial stakeholders, may be in fact seen as a violation of the rules an expert should obey. In fact, Bayesian reasoning requires the formulation of priors, in the sense that intends to measure the change of belief in something after the acquisition of new data. A popular solution to this problem suggests that the expert must adopt equal priors for both prosecution and defense. This apparently inviting solution, since it seems to respect the expert's neutrality, obliges nevertheless the expert to formulate an opinion outside his/her field of expertise. In this case, it is obviously an unpleasant hidden opinion: that *all extra-genetical evidence is absent*, or that *the prosecution has randomly chosen this person as suspect*. Those reasons seem thus more than enough to recommend the delivery of quantitative FG reports (whenever possible; in some situations, this is not feasible, as in some cases involving nonhuman materials, as shown in II.7–II.9) in the format of ratio of expected frequencies of the observations according to the two hypotheses.

Although illustrated with an example for criminalistics, the same considerations apply to all classical forensic questions, as in disputed kinships (BOX 6 and BOX 7). As before, FG cannot, strictly speaking, answer the question: *is X the father of Y?* (see II.2). An extra complication derives from the fact that frequently no biological sample of the putative father is available, and the questioned paternity is approached by collecting relatives. When that occurs, it must be clear (and explicitly indicated when reporting) that *whenever a biological sample of the questioned person X is unavailable, what is evaluated is the kinship of the ancillary relatives (assumed to be truly related biologically) of* Y. For instance, if only the parents of X are analyzed, FG will not be able to assess paternity, but 'grandparentness', i.e., the kinship of both (grandmother and grandfather) relatively to Y. It goes without saying that X can be in fact the father of Y, not being the son of their alleged parents (or of just one of them), or, maybe worse, not being the true father, can be an uncle of Y.

In conclusion, *whatever the type of forensic problem (from identification to kinship), FG is unable to contribute to an answer without the genetic profiling of the questioned individual, and the indirect approach of using relatives is problematic on genetic and ethical grounds* (BOX 20).

These limitations apply to human FG, for which standard, validated genetic markers for profiling are abundant and characterized in most populations. In case of problems involving non-human material, the situation is generally much less satisfactory, but in a quite variable degree, depending on the organisms involved (see II.6–9). In the limit, *for a completely unstudied species, whatever the type of forensic problem, FG is only able to provide answers of investigative nature and not a validated report.*

Answers without questions

Many, if not most, of the forensic questions we have discussed were literally unthinkable or deemed impossible to answer, prior to the development of techniques and theoretical developments in Genetics. These developments were rarely, if ever, driven by the purpose of applying them to solving forensic problems.

Not so long ago, it was thought to be impossible to extract relevant genetic information from most kinds of material evidence, while today even vestigial traces can be analyzed by already standard FG procedures, allowing the reliable production of genetic profiles. That tremendous increase in the analytical capacity of FG has revolutionized the strategies and procedures of evidence collection and preservation of evidence. This is particularly true in the changes of sampling at crime scene but also in wildlife forensics, missing persons identifications or even kinship assignment (e.g., non-invasive fetal typing to assess if the pregnancy results from a rape).

On the other hand, the increase in hardware and software capabilities has provided not only the analysis of highly complex problems requiring previously prohibitive computational time, but also the tackling of truly innovative questions, such as those involving distant and/or complex kinships, very often requiring the handling of massive amounts of data.

This historic experience shows that pure genetics research and FG exert a role that transcends the classical view of forensic sciences as auxiliary of justice, since they introduce changes (both at the investigative and probative phases) in the ways the litigants, prosecutors, and defense alike, design their strategies and formulate their questions to experts.

Another source of limitations to, or (conscient or not) reformulation of, forensic questions which is many times neglected, has to do with the legal and ethical framework of investigation and litigation. This framework is obviously widely different from place to place (sometimes inside the same country, particularly in federal states, as USA or Brazil) and subject to profound changes in relatively short time. Suffices to recall the recent evolution of the definition of individual rights and their limits, and how they are attributed to different citizens, according to their gender or other characteristics, to be fully aware of the dynamic nature of the societies' ethical perceptions and their reflection on the legal system.

There are therefore variable imposed or accepted limits to what, how, and in relation to whom can forensic investigations be undertaken, and consequently which questions can be posed to FG. A few examples have been given in relation to humans (BOX 15), many of them related to the difficulties of application of the 'informed consent' concept. This issue, already raised by the familial searching of forensic databases has gained more importance with the use of 'recreational' genetic databases for forensic purposes. This concept assumed the individual property of each one genetic makeup and therefore the individual right to allow (or not) its use and disclosure for any purpose, including in forensics. The trouble is that everyone's genetic makeup is nothing less than a complex sampling made on the genomes of the parents. Being so, the access to an individual genetic information permits the knowledge of genetic information from relatives of that person, a power that has allowed the identification of the authors of quite mediatic "cold cases". As recently recognized, "The consent debate incorrectly assumed that at stake was a straightforward concept of privacy — one person, making an individual choice about his or her exposure" [when indeed] it's a collective decision [Your DNA Test Could Send a Relative to Jail. https://www.nytimes.com/2021/12/27/magazine/dna-test-crime-identification-genome.html?smid=em-share]. To reach such a collective decision is utopian even for close relatives and we fear that most of those involved in the consent are not aware that their allowance involves the disclosure of significant parts of the genome of relatives, including of those who may have not granted the permission.

Another level of complexity has been recently added, by the extension of legal protection motivated by the growth of ethical concerns with non-humans. Animals are now object in many countries of specific laws aiming their well being (mainly domesticates) and protection (particularly wild species). The case of animals being the cause of offenses to humans (or property) is also to be mentioned, as it is reminiscent of the current debate on the autonomous vehicles. Traditionally, the responsibility of the offense is transferred to the owner of animal, but in many situations, the animal is not privately owned (or the owner cannot be identified). The attribution of the responsibility to the state (as when herds are attacked by wolves) or to the entity legally responsible for the area where the offense has occurred (as in traffic accidents caused by animals in highways). These attributions are however often controversial, and the liability of the animal trainers has been claimed, in a similar way to what happens with self-driving cars manufacturers.

FURTHER INFO

Amorim, A. and Pinto, N. (2018). Big data in forensic genetics. Forensic Sci. Int. Genet., 37: 102–105. doi: 10.1016/j.fsigen.2018.08.001.

Curley, L.J., Munro, J. and Dror, I.E. (2022). Cognitive and human factors in legal layperson decision making: Sources of bias in juror decision making. Med. Sci. Law., 62(3): 206–215. doi: 10.1177/00258024221080655.

Dror, I.E. (2020). Cognitive and human factors in expert decision making: Six fallacies and the eight sources of bias. Anal. Chem., 92(12): 7998–8004. doi: 10.1021/acs.analchem.0c00704.

Errickson, D., Giles, S.B. and Horsman, G. (2019). The CSI Effect(s no one?). J. Forensic Leg. Med., 67: 64–65. doi: 10.1016/j.jflm.2019.05.017.

Lidén, M. and Dror, I.E. (2021). Expert reliability in legal proceedings: "Eeny, Meeny, Miny, Moe, with which expert should we go?". Sci. Justice, 61(1): 37–46. doi: 10.1016/j.scijus.2020.09.006.

Valerio, R. (2020). Likelihood ratios for lawyers…I didn't go to law school for this! WIREs Forensic Sci., 2: e1366.

IV
Boxes

BOX 1

Biology Essentials

Cells & Reproduction

All living beings (with exception of viruses if they can be considered as living) are made up of cells. Cells are dynamic bags capable of some sort of energy usage and are endowed with genetic material (DNA), enabling them to have independent replication. The most simple and oldest cells (prokaryotes) do not have their genetic material enclosed in an inner bag, in contrast with the evolutionary more recent cells (eukaryotes), which have (most of it) enclosed in a nucleus. These eukaryotic cells are thought to be the result of fusions between prokaryotic ones. Cells of animals, plants, and fungi all possess mitochondria, which have a genetic material of their own, reproducing independently from the nucleus, and (most) plants also have plastids, another type of genetically independent structure. Therefore, eukaryotic cells have more than one genome: two or three, as shown in this plant cell ideogram:

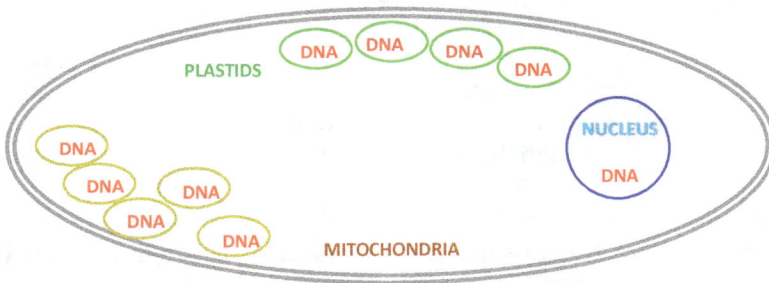

While most prokaryotes like bacteria are unicellular, many eukaryotes are multicellular and each cell keeps a semi-independent life, keeping their genetic material. So, the rule is that while unicellular organisms reproduce in a way that one individual produces two, multicellular organisms produce specialized germinal cells (gametes, containing half of the nuclear genetic material) that fuse to form an egg, a process called sexual reproduction. This egg cell will divide in multiple rounds to form a new multicellular individual, now by asexual reproduction. So, in the sexual reproduction of multicellular organisms, two individuals produce one, but their individual body (somatic) growth and development are done by asexual cellular reproduction. Using our species case as an example:

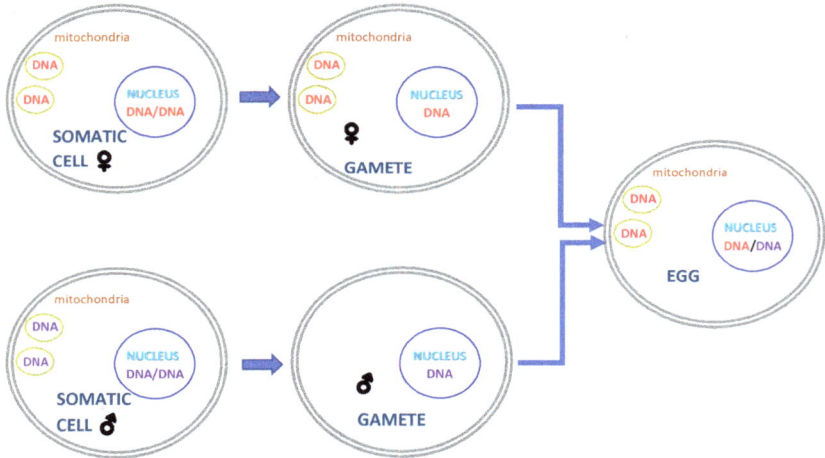

The development of an egg into a multicellular organism can be disturbed, and a single egg can be divided and grow independently into two or more genetically identical individuals (monozygotic twins) or, symmetrically, two or more eggs may fuse into a single individual, creating a chimera. Chimerism can also result from later events, such as transfusion, transplantation, or pregnancy (foetus cells may be present in the mother's body after birth). Genetic heterogeneity among cells from the same individual can also arise from copy errors when replicating DNA (mutations) in dividing body (somatic) cells, a situation called mosaicism. So even monozygotic twins, although germinally identical, do accumulate differences, which increase with age. Contrasting with germinal mutations, occurring in the formation of gametes, somatic mutations are not transmitted to offspring. Many multicellular organisms (including those from sexual reproduction) are capable of **clonal** reproduction, detaching part of the body to form a new individual (as twinning above, but in the adult stage).

BOX 2

Genetics

The genetic information in all living beings (except for viruses, if they can be considered as living) is encoded in DNA, as explained in BOX 1. Nevertheless, the ways that DNA is preserved, copied, and inherited vary a lot, not only among organisms, but also inside the same organism, corresponding to quite distinct patterns, or modes of transmission.

The simplest mode of transmission is observed regularly in prokaryotic organisms and somatic cells of multicellular organisms: the DNA of the progenitor cell is duplicated and divided equally into daughter cells. In this clonal mode of transmission, the only source of novelty is the occurrence of DNA copy errors (mutations), and unless this occurs, the genetic parental and filial information will be similar.

In eukaryotic multicellular organisms, DNA is organized in different cell compartments and their mode of transmission to individual descendants also varies. By far, the greater fraction is stored in the cell nucleus and packed into pairs of independently transmitting structures (chromosomes), each member of the same pair containing homologous information from both parents (i.e., coding for the same external characteristic of the organism). That pairing rule has a notable exception: in many species, as for humans, sex is determined by sex chromosomes. Exemplified by *Homo sapiens*, in our body cells the nuclear genomic library is packed into 23 pairs of ordinary (autosomal) chromosomes in females, while males possess 22 of these autosomes, plus a heterogeneous pseudo pair, containing a chromosome identical to the one observed in females (X chromosome) and a much smaller one (Y chromosome). So, while all the female nuclear genome is diploid, a part of it in males is not, leading to a situation called haplodiploidy: diploid XX in females and haploid X in males. Males can produce two types of gametes (they are heterogametic): those carrying an X and determining the female sex of a resulting egg and those with Y, which will determine a male.

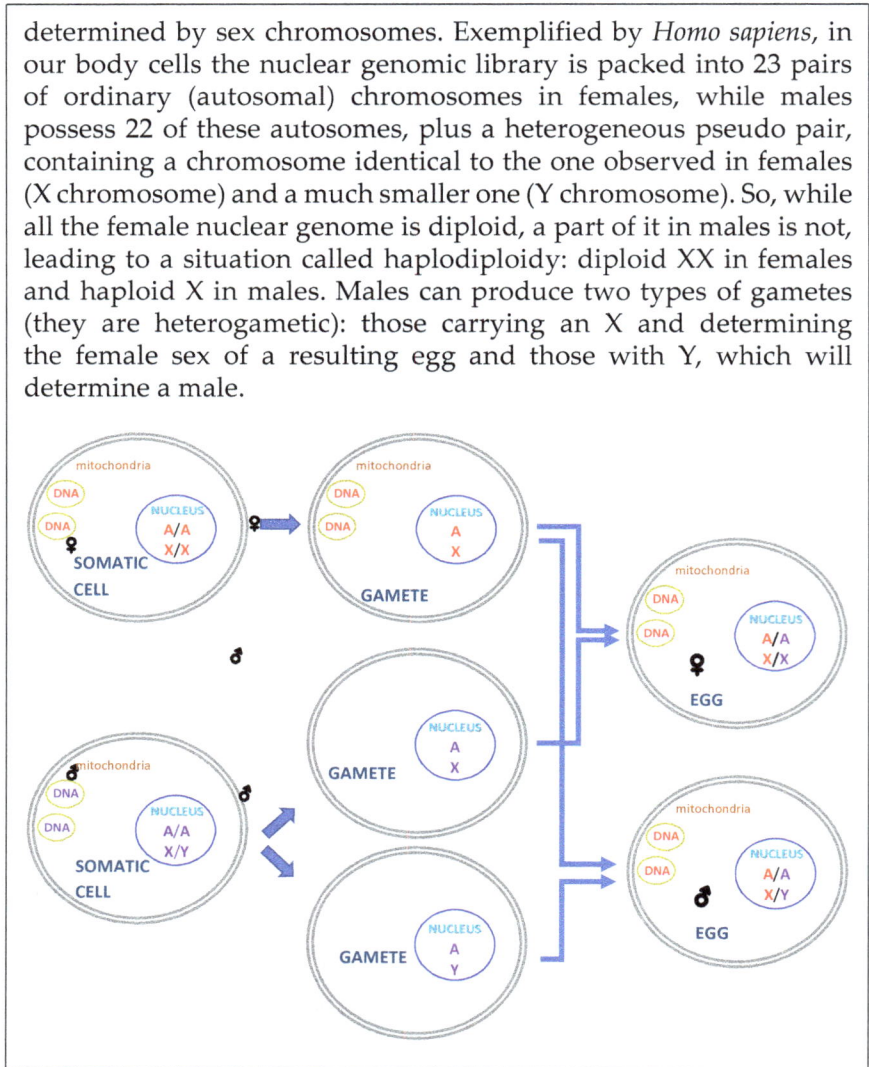

BOX 3

Genetic Markers

Current techniques allow the analysis of the entire genetic makeup of a cell (although with some limitations and pitfalls, particularly in their forensic use). Nevertheless, the established and validated genetic analyses use limited and well-defined zones of a genome (locus, plural loci) as genetic markers. Both the definition and the kind of information retrieved from these targeted regions, as well as the success and reliability of the obtained results, depend therefore on the technical approach employed.

Most routine methods used in Forensic Genetics for analyzing genetic markers rely on a preanalytical step which consists in the specific amplification of DNA from a previously studied region of the genome (a locus), by PCR (Polymerase Chain Reaction). This technique is able to produce, out of vestigial samples, many copies of the aimed locus, DNA which is sufficient to be submitted to subsequent analysis.

This technology was therefore revolutionary, in allowing the genetic analysis of material evidence in which the DNA quantity content is far below the detection threshold for direct typing. However, the use of PCR introduces complexities and adds sources of errors when analyzing results, which a layperson must be aware of when using these results to ground decisions. Here we will consider the analyses error-free, and we will limit our discussion to the formal analyses of the results (which can also be of quite different technical nature, with correspondingly diverse problems; see BOX 13).

Once a genetic marker is discovered, it will have forensic relevance only if, through some defined method, differences between individuals can be disclosed. Each alternative version of the DNA composition, observed at the same locus, is called an allele. The number of copies per cell of a locus (called ploidy) depends on the mode of transmission and the type of cell. In the loci of diploid, homogametic or autosomal transmission (BOX 5), gametes are haploid (i.e., contain just one allele per locus), whereas in our diploid body cells two copies exist, either having equal or distinct alleles (BOX 2). In the diploid cells of an individual, it may happen that identical alleles are present at a certain locus and then the individual is said to be a homozygote at that locus, while at a different locus, two different alleles are present and then the individual is a heterozygote for the latter locus. The allelic state of a locus in an individual corresponds to the genotype. These states are symbolized as follows: supposing a locus A with alleles A_1, A_2, A_3, ..., a homozygote for the A_1 allele is denoted by A_1A_1, while a heterozygote for alleles A_1 and A_3 is denoted by A_1A_3 (by convention, heterozygotes are always denoted in allelic symbol order). Below is depicted one X chromosomal locus (DXS10101) amplified in two females carrying the genotypes 30–31 (left, heterozygous) and 30.2–30.2 (right, homozygous assuming the absence of silent alleles–BOX 13).

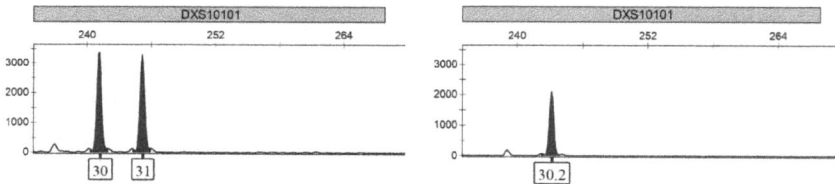

Forensic analyses routinely aim at various genetic markers at the same time, so it usually happens that an individual is typed as a heterozygote at some loci and homozygote at others.

The following table allows a first glimpse at the amount of information that can be obtained from these analyses and how it grows with the number of alleles per locus and genetic markers, typed in a diploid species like ours. A more quantified view on the forensic informative power will be possible when dealing with allele frequency distribution in the population (BOX 9; BOX 14).

Locus	Number of		Genetic profiles
	Alleles	**Genotypes**	
A	2	3	homozygotes A_1A_1, A_2A_2, heterozygote A_1A_2
B	3	6	homozygotes A_1A_1, A_2A_2, A_3A_3 heterozygotes A_1A_2, A_1A_3, A_2A_3
C	4	10	homozygotes A_1A_1, A_2A_2, A_3A_3, A_4A_4 heterozygotes A_1A_2, A_1A_3, A_1A_4, A_2A_3, A_2A_4, A_3A_4
D	5	15	homozygotes A_1A_1, A_2A_2, A_3A_3, A_4A_4, A_5A_5 heterozygotes A_1A_2, A_1A_3, A_1A_4, A_1A_5, A_2A_3, A_2A_4, A_2A_5, A_3A_4, A_3A_5, A_4A_5
Combined	–	2700	Nearly 3 thousand

BOX 4

Genetics Theory

Genetics was founded and theorized well before the acceptance of DNA as a carrier of the hereditary information and the advent of technological advances allowing its analysis. At that time, only visible characteristics were available to infer what genetic properties would be responsible for the observed variations. Therefore, the conceptual framework in which genetic theory was developed is based on this inferential paradigm and is still used today. The theory advanced by Mendel in 1865 limits its field of application to discrete, discontinuous variations observed as a specific feature among the members of the same species, so that individuals can be unambiguously classified into well-defined groups or types. Classical human ABO blood groups are a good example: Under a specific observational protocol, individuals are grouped into four classes or phenotypes (A, B, AB, and O). The question that may now arise is how these phenotypes correlate with the genetic background of the individuals. This correlation is easier to establish (and explain) using another, simpler, blood group: the Rh, factor D, for which each individual has only two possible phenotypes: positive or negative. In controlled family studies, it was verified that when parents are both negative (phenotype symbol d), all offspring are invariably negative, while positive descendants were observed in all other types of couples, namely in the case of both parents being positive (phenotype symbol: D). These apparently contradictory observations, suggesting on one hand that the characteristic is hereditary (all offspring from **d** couples are also **d**), or the contrary (parents **D** may have **d** children), is solved if we assume that the information coding for **d** can be hidden in individuals **D**, nonetheless being able to be transmitted. That is why the two alternative types of genetic information responsible for the observable characteristic (alleles) are symbolized accordingly as d, for the allele that can be hidden (and called recessive), and **D** for the dominant. The global genetic interpretation for the Rh marker is the following:

Phenotype	Genotype
d	dd
D	DD or Dd

Mating type	Offspring		
	Genotype	Phenotype	Probability
DD × DD	DD	D	1
DD × Dd	DD	D	½
	Dd	D	½
DD × dd	Dd	D	1
Dd × Dd	DD	D	¼
	Dd	D	½
	dd	d	¼
Dd × dd	Dd	D	½
	dd	d	½
dd × dd	dd	d	1

			Mother Dd gametes	
			½ D	½ d
Father Dd	gametes	½ D	¼ DD	¼ Dd
		½ d	¼ Dd	¼ dd

For the ABO system, phenotype/genotype correlation is more complex, since both A and B alleles are dominant over O, but **codominant** between them:

Phenotype	Genotype
A	AA or AO
B	BB or BO
AB	AB
O	OO

The theory, in its original form, proposes then that there are two alleles at each diploid loci in each individual, but only one, chosen at random (hence, the probability of ½) is passed to the offspring. It further hypothesizes that if the transmissions of two (or more) loci are studied simultaneously, the gametes combine freely at random.

We now know that there are other possibilities, and the Mendelian theory has been generalized to incorporate association between loci, that is, the genetic information observed for one specific locus is not independent of the one at another locus, as well as other rules of transmission, namely sex linkage. Anyway, in FG, this is the central model and when nothing is explicitly specified, the diploid genetic markers employed obey these transmission rules.

BOX 5

Transmission Modes

All the genetic information is encoded in DNA, which is organized and distributed in diverse forms inside the cells of the complex organisms so that, when cells divide and organisms reproduce, DNA transmission rules are also heterogeneous (BOX 1 and BOX 2).

We will not examine this variety of transmission modes across the tree of life, but just those occurring inside the same species, choosing a well-studied one: *Homo sapiens*. This means that we will study the transmission of the genetic markers located at the nucleus of the human cells, including at sex chromosomes, as well as those located in mitochondria.

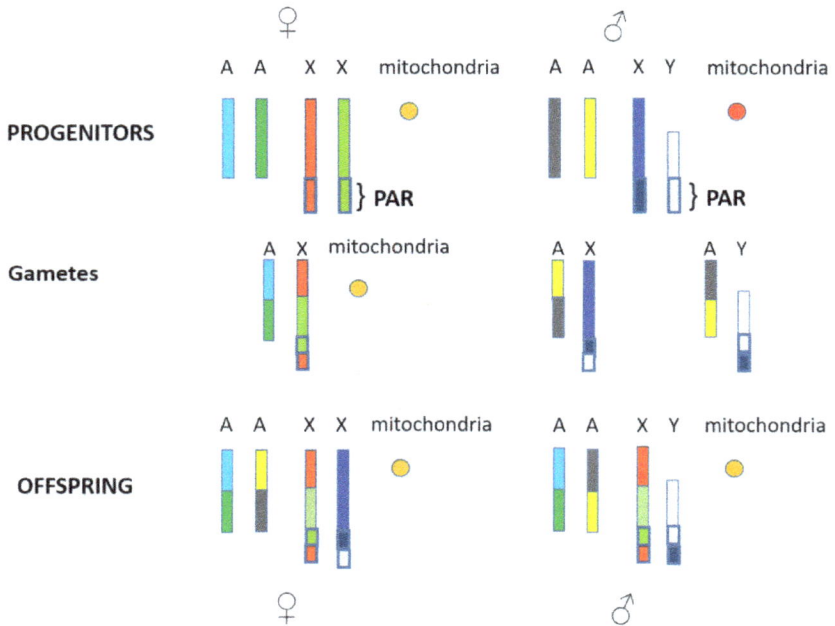

Beginning with the extranuclear DNA, which in our species is limited to mitochondria (mtDNA, a circular molecule as depicted), we see that it is transmitted exclusively by the mother (to both sons and daughters).

The rest of the cells' DNA is organized in linear form, hence the bars—each symbolizing a chromosome. Only the sex chromosomes (X and Y) and one pair out of the remnant chromosomal set (autosomes, which are 22) are shown (labelled A).

The genetic behavior of an autosomal locus is exactly the one predicted by Mendelian theory in its original form, as well as when studying two (or more) markers if they are located at different pairs (i.e., they are independently transmitted). However, if located closely in the same chromosome, they are not independently transmitted, or in other words, they do not recombine freely. That is depicted in the scheme above by the colors used for chromosome A: for instance, in the female progenitor, blue and green (one received from her mother and the other from the father). The resulting gamete bears a bicolored chromosome, meaning that markers in the blue region (maternal origin) are rearranged (recombination) with markers at the green one, but not all of them.

The largest part (the scheme does not intend to represent the proportions) of Y chromosome is transmitted in a way (almost) symmetrical to mtDNA: it is only present in males, so it is exclusively transmitted from fathers to sons (and sons only).

The label PAR at the end of Y chromosome depicts a part of it that is homologous to the X chromosome (hence the name: Pseudo Autosomal Region; humans indeed have two, one at each chromosomal tip, but only one is represented in the scheme for simplicity reasons). Genetic markers at PAR behave (almost) as the autosomal described above.

Last, but not least, the X chromosome has a very peculiar situation as it is present in two copies in females and just one in males. In the females, the pair of X chromosomes behave just like the autosomes, while in males the X chromosome is transmitted to the daughters (and daughters only, never to sons). In summary, depending on their location, human genetic markers can follow four modes of genetic transmission (BOX 5): haploid or uniparental (maternal – mtDNA, or paternal – Y chromosome specific), diploid (homogametic – autosomal chromosomes), or haplodiploid (heterogametic – X chromosome).

BOX 6

Genealogies and Kinships

In many instances, the purpose of FG is to genetically validate some genealogy or a specific kinship between individuals. Given the diverse modes of transmission of the genetic information existing in complex organisms, these apparently simple and univocally meaning concepts gain different perspectives, according to the type of genetic markers employed. We will again use the example of *Homo sapiens*, assuming that we have typed all the members of this genealogy for forensically validated genetic markers — one at an autosomal chromosome, (A, diploid), two at the sex chromosomes (one Y specific, haploid, parentally transmitted, and one X specific, haplodiploid, heterogametic), and one at mtDNA (haploid, maternally transmitted), depicting all the modes of transmission in humans. The superscripts represent allelic states found.

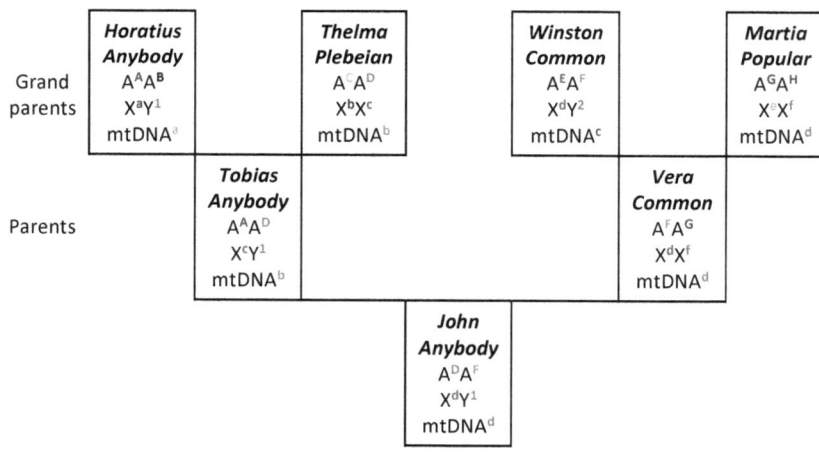

	Horatius Anybody $A^A A^B$ $X^a Y^1$ $mtDNA^a$		Thelma Plebeian $A^C A^D$ $X^b X^c$ $mtDNA^b$		Winston Common $A^E A^F$ $X^d Y^2$ $mtDNA^c$		Martia Popular $A^G A^H$ $X^e X^f$ $mtDNA^d$
Grand parents							
Parents		Tobias Anybody $A^A A^D$ $X^c Y^1$ $mtDNA^b$				Vera Common $A^F A^G$ $X^d X^f$ $mtDNA^d$	
			John Anybody $A^D A^F$ $X^d Y^1$ $mtDNA^d$				

82

Analyzing the transmission genetic markers, we observe that John's:

- mtDNA^d came from Vera (his mother) who in turn, received it from Martia (his maternal grandmother);

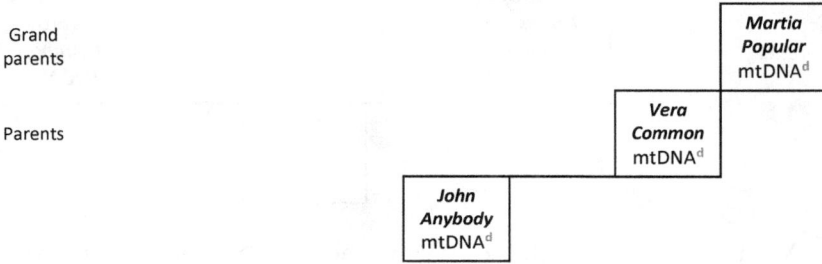

Grand parents		**Martia** *Popular* mtDNA^d
	Vera *Common* mtDNA^d	
Parents		
John *Anybody* mtDNA^d		

- Y^1 came from Tobias (his father) who in turn, received it from Horatius (his paternal grandfather);

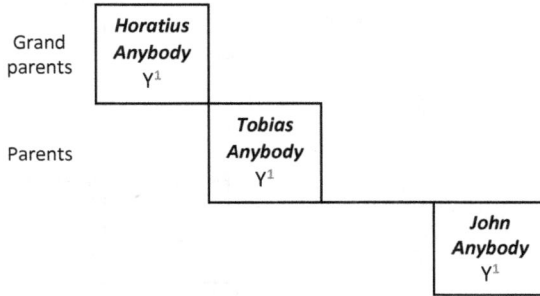

Grand parents	**Horatius** *Anybody* Y^1	
	Tobias *Anybody* Y^1	
Parents		
		John *Anybody* Y^1

- A^D came from Tobias (his father) who in turn, received it from Thelma (his paternal grandmother, and A^F came from Vera (his mother) who in turn, received it from Winston (his maternal grandfather);

83

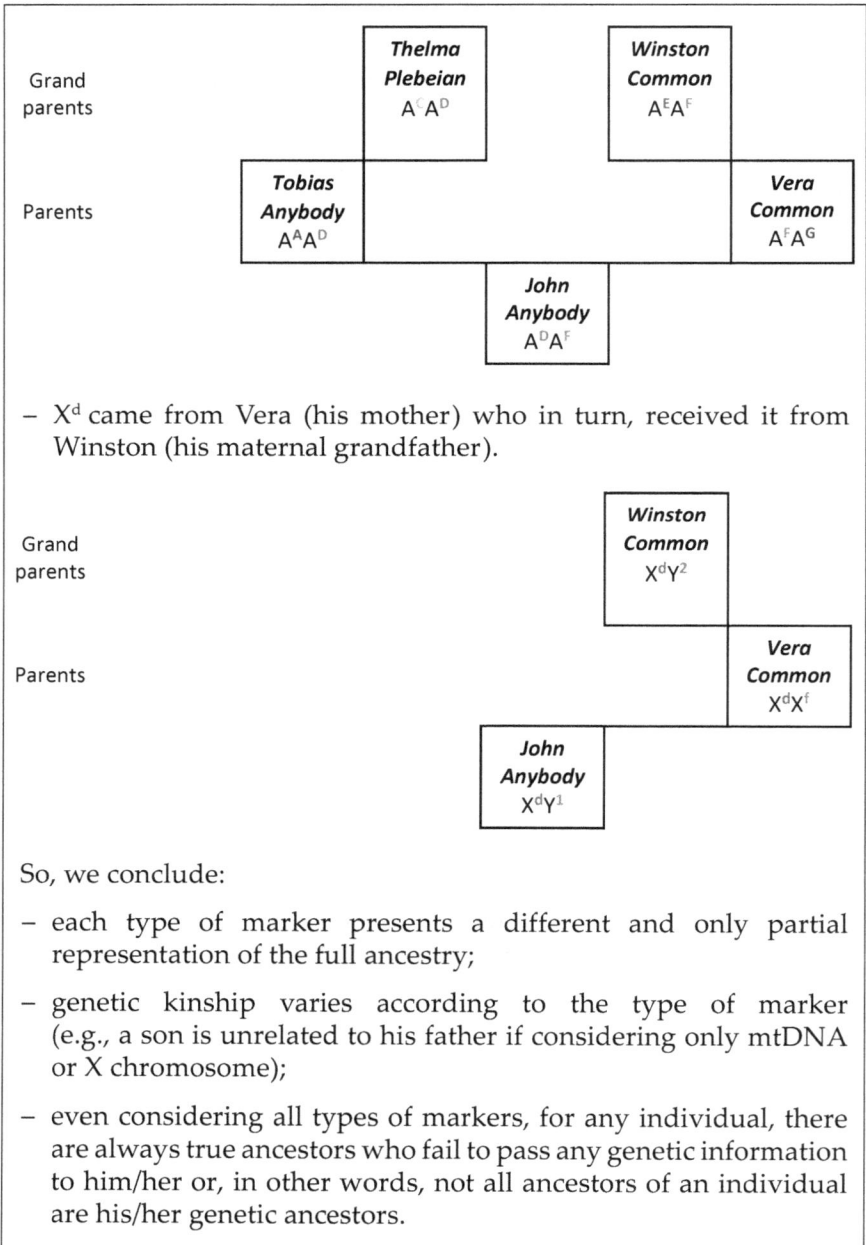

Grand parents		**Thelma Plebeian** $A^C A^D$		**Winston Common** $A^E A^F$	
Parents	**Tobias Anybody** $A^A A^D$				**Vera Common** $A^F A^G$
			John Anybody $A^D A^F$		

- X^d came from Vera (his mother) who in turn, received it from Winston (his maternal grandfather).

Grand parents				**Winston Common** $X^d Y^2$	
Parents					**Vera Common** $X^d X^f$
			John Anybody $X^d Y^1$		

So, we conclude:

- each type of marker presents a different and only partial representation of the full ancestry;

- genetic kinship varies according to the type of marker (e.g., a son is unrelated to his father if considering only mtDNA or X chromosome);

- even considering all types of markers, for any individual, there are always true ancestors who fail to pass any genetic information to him/her or, in other words, not all ancestors of an individual are his/her genetic ancestors.

BOX 7

Kinships - Classification and Quantification

From the genetics point of view, two individuals are said to be related if the probability of sharing at least one allele (↑Glossary) from a common ancestor is greater than zero. These alleles are called identical-by-descent (or IBD) and ground the theory of the classification and quantification of genetic kinships between individuals. Indeed, considering some point in the past beyond which individuals are assumed to be unrelated, the weighing of any kin link existing between two individuals is based on the probabilities of sharing IBD alleles. One individual whose parents are related is said to be inbred and may carry two IBD alleles at the same locus (↑Glossary).

Given an autosomal locus (BOX 5) and a pair of non-inbred individuals, there are three possibilities for IBD allele sharing, as they may share none, one, or two pairs of IBD alleles—k_0, k_1, and k_2, respectively. If considering the possibility of inbred individuals, the number of possible IBD autosomal patterns increases from three to nine—Δ_1 to Δ_9 as depicted in the scheme below, in which each dot represents one allele, and each set of four dots represents the four alleles of the individuals I_1 (the two at the top) and I_2 (the two at the bottom); two dots are linked if, and only if, they are IBD alleles. Note that in the first two lines (from Δ_1 to Δ_6), either I_1 or I_2 or both are inbred (which is represented by a horizontal line connecting alleles from the same individual), whereas in the last line (from Δ_7 to Δ_9) both I_1 and I_2 are not inbred (absence of horizontal connections). Inbred or not, I_1 and I_2 can be related (which is represented by vertical line connecting alleles from different individuals) as in the cases of Δ_7 and Δ_8 but not in Δ_9. In the case of autosomal markers, these IBD patterns are also known as Jacquard's coefficients.

Δ_1 I_1: • —— • Δ_2 I_1: • —— • Δ_3 I_1: • —— •

I_2: • —— • I_2: • —— • I_2: • •

Δ_4 I_1: • —— • Δ_5 I_1: • • Δ_6 I_1: • •

I_2: • • I_2: • —— • I_2: • —— •

$\Delta_7 (k_2)$ I_1: • • $\Delta_8 (k_1)$ I_1: • • $\Delta_9 (k_0)$ I_1: • •

I_2: • • I_2: • • I_2: • •

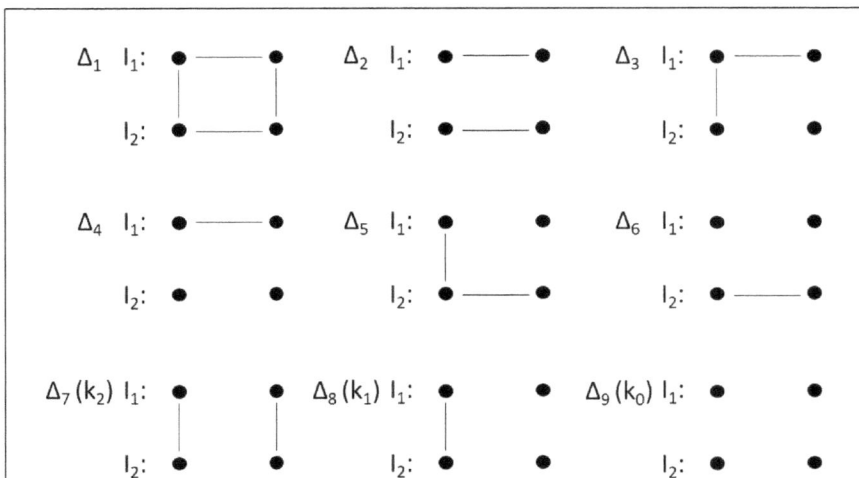

The IBD patterns describe any genetic relationship existing between a pair of individuals and are independent of the genotypes of the individuals.

Unless mutation, two IBD alleles are also identical by state (or IBS); the reciprocal not being true. For example, in a standard paternity test where the individuals share one allele at each marker, what is evaluated is the possibility of such alleles being similar by inheritance (individuals related as parent-child) or by mere chance (unrelated individuals).

There are only three relationships for which the probability of sharing exactly either two, one, or zero pairs of IBD alleles for any marker equates 100%, which are monozygotic twins (↑Glossary), parent-child, and unrelated individuals, respectively. For all the other relationships, individuals may or may not share IBD alleles. For example, a pair of full siblings may share *(i)* two pairs of IBD alleles (25%), if they have received the same maternal and paternal alleles, *(ii)* one pair of IBD alleles (50%), if they received the same maternal allele and a different paternal one, or vice versa, and *(iii)* none pair of IBD alleles (25%), if they received different alleles from both the mother and the father. In other words, we can say that, for a single marker, a pair of full siblings is related as a pair of monozygotic twins, parent-child, and unrelated individuals with corresponding probabilities of 25%, 50%, and 25%, respectively. In the case of half-siblings, the probability of sharing two pairs of IBD alleles is null—as they do not share one of the parents, while it is equally likely for the individuals sharing one or none pair of IBD alleles, considering the genetic transmission from the sole common parent. In other words, it is equally likely a pair of half-siblings being related as either a parent-child or unrelated. The same reasoning can be applied for more distant pedigrees. For example, a pair of cousins, offspring of two full brothers (mothers unrelated), shares for a specific autosomal marker one pair of IBD alleles (inherited from one of the two common grandparents) with a probability of 25%. The same individuals are not able to share two pairs of IBD alleles as their mothers are unrelated, and thus they do not share any pair of IBD alleles with 75% of probability. A greater genetic proximity is obviously expected if the mothers of the individuals are also related, e.g., as full-sisters—double first cousins—in which case the individuals have four common grandparents and may share two pairs of IBD alleles at an autosomal locus. If the cousins are offspring of a pair of half-siblings, the genetic proximity is of course smaller, reducing the probability of the individuals sharing a pair of IBD alleles to 12.5%.

We hope to have shown with these examples that the accurate formulation of the genetic kinships is crucial for their proper mathematical treatment and statistical evaluation. Indeed, the algebraic formulae needed to weigh the probabilities of the observations given the alternative hypotheses, compared via a likelihood ratio (BOX 14), fully depend on these IBD parameters and on the population frequencies of alleles and mutation events (BOX 9), as well as on other characteristics of the population.

On the other hand, it should be clearly remarked that *different kinships may have the same IBD patterns, which implies that they are theoretically indistinguishable from the genetical point of view when using only autosomal markers.* This is, for example, the case of pedigrees such as grandparent-grandchild, half-siblings, and avuncular, regardless of the number of independent autosomal markers analyzed. Pedigrees with the same IBD partitions associated, and therefore indistinguishable, are said to belong to the same kinship class. In practical terms, this can be relevant in a plethora of cases. Suppose, for example, that both the grandson G and the nephew N of an individual X are missing, and an anatomically uninformative part of a body was recovered nearby. If only the individual X is available for analysis, it is *a priori* known that it is useless to analyze unlinked autosomal markers as the probabilities of the observations assuming the unidentified part of the body belong to either G or N are the same.

IBD partitions can be established for all the modes of genetic transmission, implying that *the same pedigree carries different levels of genetics similarity* (and IBD partition patterns) *depending on the type of transmission mode* of the analyzed markers. Consider, for example, a father-son pair. From the point of view of the Y chromosomal transmission, and unless there is mutation, these individuals are identical, sharing 100% of the alleles. Considering autosomal transmission, genetic similarity by common ancestry reduces to 50%, as exactly one of the two pairs of the alleles of the individuals are IBD. Finally, considering X-chromosomal and mtDNA markers, the inherited similarity is absent (0%), and the father-son pair behaves as a pair of unrelated individuals (again assuming that the son is not inbred, i.e., that the father is not related to the mother).

The fact that different modes of transmission carry different levels of informativeness has practical forensic implications in kinship problems. For example, when two females are questioned to be related either as paternal half-sisters or as unrelated, autosomal markers may provide very little information, as there is a 50% of chance they do not share IBD alleles (as unrelated individuals). Notwithstanding, powerful results are expected when considering X chromosomal markers since two paternal half-sisters must share the paternal allele for any marker.

FURTHER INFO

Egeland, T., Pinto, N. and Vigeland, M. (2014). A general approach to power calculation for relationship testing. Forensic Sci. Int. Genet., 9: 186–90. doi: 10.1016/j.fsigen.2013.05.001.

Gonçalves, J., Conde-Sousa, E., Egeland, T., Amorim, A. and Pinto, N. (2017). Key individuals for discerning pedigrees belonging to the same autosomal kinship class. Forensic Sci. Int. Genet., 29: 71–79. doi: 10.1016/j.fsigen.2017.03.018.

Pinto, N., Gusmão, L. and Amorim, A. (2010). Likelihood ratios in kinship analysis: Contrasting kinship classes, not genealogies. Forensic Sci. Int. Genet., 4(3): 218–9. doi: 10.1016/j.fsigen.2009.06.010.

Pinto, N., Gusmão, L. and Amorim, A. (2011). X-chromosome markers in kinship testing: A generalisation of the IBD approach identifying situations where their contribution is crucial. Forensic Sci. Int. Genet., 5(1): 27–32. doi: 10.1016/j.fsigen.2010.01.011.

Pinto, N., Gusmão, L., Egeland, T. and Amorim, A. (2013). Paternity exclusion power: Comparative behaviour of autosomal and X-chromosomal markers in standard and deficient cases with inbreeding. Forensic Sci. Int. Genet., 7(2): 290-5. doi: 10.1016/j.fsigen.2012.12.002.

Weir, B.S., Anderson, A.D. and Hepler, A.B. (2006). Genetic relatedness analysis: Modern data and new challenges. Nat. Rev. Genet., 7(10): 771–80. doi: 10.1038/nrg1960. Erratum in: Nat. Rev. Genet., 23(2): 134.

BOX 8

Population Genetics

Genetics theory was initially formulated at the family level, allowing researchers to predict the genotypic structure of the offspring given the parents' genotypes, or conversely, knowing the offspring genotypes, to infer the possible genotypes of the parents. In that form, it only works with one-generation kinships and when the genotypic structure of either the parental or the descendent generation is (at least partially) known. To address the genotypic structure (in probability terms) of unrelated individuals, it was necessary to extend the theory to the population level. That was made using quite a simple model of a population, usually known as the **Hardy-Weinberg (HW)** formalism. This model assumes that the population has an infinite size and the members mate at random with respect to the genotype (a **panmictic population**). It further assumes an absence of mutation (↑BOX 1), migration, and selection (no reproductive differences between genotypes). From this simple model (which can be generalized to other modes of transmission and to different assumptions), it is quite simple to infer allele frequencies from the observed genotype (or phenotype) distributions.

Using the Rh blood group example (↑BOX 4), the relation between these two variables can be seen in the following scheme (p and q = 1–p, stand for the allele frequencies of D and d, respectively), in which the gamete (allele or gene) pool is sampled randomly to produce new individuals (sex is irrelevant in the homogametic mode of transmission ↑BOX 5):

		gametes	
		p	q
		D	d
gametes	p D	p^2 DD	pq Dd
	q d	pq Dd	q^2 dd

Or, algebraically:

$$(p+q)^2 = p^2 + 2pq + q^2$$

That is, it means that the expected frequency of Rh negative individuals (genotype dd) is the square of the allele frequency q, or, inversely, that we can estimate the frequency of the Rh negative allele q, as the square root of the observed frequency of Rh negative individuals.

Further, we can also unveil, among phenotypically indistinguishable Rh+ individuals, the proportions corresponding to DD and Dd genotypes.

The generalization to the analysis of two or more markers is straightforward, provided they are not associated, that is, the allelic state of one marker is independent of that of other markers. For example, if dealing with two markers (A and B, with alleles A1, A2, and B1, B2), there will be four types of gametes (A1B1, A1B2, A2B1, and A2B2). As markers A and B are independent, an individual having the allele A1 in marker A does not provide any information on the allele present in marker B. The frequencies of each of these gametes equate to the product of the frequencies of the genes involved. For instance, if the frequency of A1 is p and of B1 u, the frequency of the gamete A1B1 will be p×u. Then, the expected frequency of A1B1/A1B1 individuals is $(pu)^2$.

Note that to the HW assumptions for single marker analysis, we are adding the requirement of absence of association between markers. This simple model can be extended to situations where an association between markers does exist, that is, the allelic information at one marker is not independent of the one at another marker. For the same example above, if one individual has the allele A1 at marker A, it can be more (or less) likely he/she has the allele B1 at marker B, instead of allele B2. In this case, calculations are much more complex and require the estimation of extra parameters, which are exceedingly difficult to ascertain with precision.

The markers used in forensics are evaluated before entering into practical use, which includes the analysis of the frequencies of the respective alleles and genotypes in different populations. To simplify calculations, allowing the simple product of frequencies, associated diploid markers are avoided. This is not possible if we use linked markers (such as those of mtDNA or Y chromosome), several markers (> 4) located in the same chromosome (as those from the X chromosome), or a very large number of markers (viz., a genome-wide approach).

BOX 9

Statistics
Parameters and Estimates

The genetics theory underlying all the forensically relevant calculations of expected frequencies requires the knowledge of the values of some parameters, such as allele (↑Glossary) frequencies (BOX 8). These values are estimated in the population of interest by randomly sampling a desirably large number of individuals (typically several hundreds). These estimates are therefore approximations of the true value of the parameter and are subject to uncertainty regarding their precision and accuracy, and of course are limited to the sampled population.

Since frequencies may vary between populations, the definition of the relevant population in the case under analysis is an important issue. In fact, what would be appropriate to consider as the universe of potential perpetrators of a specific crime, or the universe of possible fathers in a paternity investigation? The current practice is to use a population sample from an administrative/politically defined geographical area, such as an entire country or a region inside it. In an era of great population mobility and migration, this solution poses many questions, since the genetic composition of the population may change very rapidly and the perpetrator of the crime, or the father in question, can be persons from a genetically very different population but who happened to be there at the time of the crime perpetration or the child's conception.

Although theoretically important, these difficulties are of minor impact on the final quantification of the evidence, provided the genetic markers used in forensics are in a reasonable number (typically over 15) and are those included in routinely employed commercial genotyping kits. Indeed, these markers are very diverse when considering individuals from the same population but differentiate populations very poorly. In other words, the use of an inappropriate database (i.e., from a 'wrong' population) does not significantly modify the final value of the expected frequency of a genetic profile, and overestimations committed at some of the markers are compensated by underestimations occurring at others. This especially applies to the cases of identification and paternity/maternity, where allele sharing is mandatory. The cases involving more distant pedigrees may be more sensitive to the database used.

This reassuring conclusion, that is, that the combination of various independent markers minimizes the error, is however limited to the genetic markers with a mode of transmission that is not sex-linked nor uniparental (BOX 5), for which, besides other limitations vis-à-vis identification, the rarity of the profiles poses more serious problems. The rarity of an event is a universal statistical problem and the way to deal with it is subject to controversies. Many experts advise the use of an upper limit value, for the sake of not risking to excessively burden the defense or privilege the accusation, but this opinion is not generally shared and is difficult to explain in a court environment.

Three particular types of problems raised by the rarity of events deserve some analysis: *(i)* the observation, in the case under analysis, of a previously undetected allele; *(ii)* silent alleles (↑Glossary), and *(iii)* mutation (↑Glossary).

The first is easily accommodated by adding the previously unobserved allele to the database; the estimate of its value could be simply $1/(N+1)$, N being the total number of alleles of the preexisting database, which means that the larger the database, the rarer is the event.

Silent alleles are a more serious problem, due to their recessiveness (↑Glossary) and rarity, so the estimation of their frequency is not possible by simple counting as only homozygous individuals express their presence. To estimate the frequency of silent alleles, we must therefore resort to the statistically more demanding approach of detecting transmission incompatibilities in biologically confirmed

93

families or mother/child duos (e.g., the observation: mother **A1** and child **A2**, can be interpreted as mother hiding the silent allele **s**—being **A1s**, and passed it to the child **A2s**, who received **A2** from the father). Even for laboratories having the possibility of (and being allowed to) typing this ethically sensitive material, the detection of silent genes is difficult, and most of these genes with a frequency below 0.5% go unnoticed.

Mutations, being in general rarer are still more difficult to detect and estimate their rate. Again, their detection depends on the observation of a different type of violation of transmission rules in controlled families such as mother **A1A2**/child **A3A4**, in which the child shows two alleles that are absent from the mother. Additionally, the possibility of hidden mutations, that is, mutations that do not result in incompatibilities, increases the difficulty of its frequency estimation. For example, in a duo mother **A1A2**/ child **A2A3**, we cannot be sure that the allele **A2** in the child was inherited from the mother, as a mutation **A2** (or **A1**) to **A3** may have occurred.

In any case, for the markers included in commercial kits, the average rate of mutation per marker is estimated to be around 1/1000.

FURTHER INFO

Amorim, A. and Carneiro, J. (2008). The impact of silent alleles in kinship probability calculations. Forensic Science International: Genetics Supplement Series, 1: 638–639.

Antão-Sousa, S., Conde-Sousa, E., Gusmão, L., Amorim, A. and Pinto, N. Estimations of mutation rates depend on population allele frequency distribution: The case of autosomal microsatellites. Genes (Basel)., 13(7): 1248. doi: 10.3390/genes13071248.

Laurent, F.X., Fischer, A., Oldt, R.F., Kanthaswamy, S., Buckleton, J.S. and Hitchin, S. (2022). Streamlining the decision-making process for international DNA kinship matching using Worldwide allele frequencies and tailored cutoff log10LR thresholds. Forensic Sci. Int. Genet., 57: 102634. Doi: 10.1016/j.fsigen.2021.102634.

Steele, C.D. and Balding, D.J. (2014). Choice of population database for forensic DNA profile analysis. Sci. Justice., 54(6): 487–93. doi: 10.1016/j.scijus.2014.10.004.

BOX 10

Transmission Errors
Mutations

Although the fidelity of the transmission of genetic information between parents and offspring is, in general, exceptionally high, meaning that both the structure and contents of our genome are well preserved in reproduction, some copying errors (germinal mutations ↑Glossary, BOX 1) do occur, although at a low rate individually.

These mutations can thus lead to (*i*) structural changes, in which the organization of the genetic material is altered, by simple rearrangement or variation in the number of copies; or (*ii*) by modifications of the composition of the genetic information, keeping its length unmodified. Since most of the commercial kits used for human forensic genetics use a technology that detects only the length variation of specific genetic markers, all mutations of the second type are not detected. In the following examples, the first two mutations are therefore detected while the last two go unnoticed. In the scheme, the fictitious sequences are shown as ordered rows of letters (using the DNA alphabet: A, C, G, and T).

Original DNA sequence	Altered DNA sequence	Type of mutation
CAGACAGAGT	CAGACAGA	Structural (deletion)
	CAGACAGACAGAGT	Structural (duplication)
	TGAGACAGAC	Structural (inversion)
	CAGACAGAGA	Substitution

95

The frequency of occurrence of mutations varies substantially with many factors related to the individual (such as age, sex, or environmental conditions), but also with the location and DNA sequence. For example, mtDNA (↑Glossary, BOX 1) is more mutable than the main genome, as well as some specific sequences or regions.

Genetic theory (↑Glossary BOX 4) can accommodate these events, incorporating in the calculation of expected values a rating factor related to the error transmission. However, in FG context, if we observe a genetic incompatibility, for instance, between a putative father and child that cannot be explained by the presence of a silent allele (↑Glossary, BOX 4), we can interpret the violation of the theoretical transmission rules as being attributable to either (*i*) mutation or (*ii*) false kinship.

In consequence, these incompatibilities cannot be used as qualitative evidence of paternity exclusion, but quantitatively evaluated comparatively with their expected frequencies according to the two alternative explanations.

BOX 11

Intra- and Interindividual Genetic Heterogeneity

Twins, Mosaics, and Chimeras

We are familiar with the saying that any two individuals can safely be genetically distinguished since they display significantly different genetic profiles, identical twins excepted. This knowledge of the enormous genetic diversity of individuals among sexually reproducing organisms is however not accompanied by an identical awareness of the possibility of *the same individual having more than one very distinct genetic profile.*

Indeed, not only humans but also most organisms analyzed in FG are complex and the sexual mode of reproduction is the rule among them (BOX 1). Despite the complexity and multicellularity of the organisms, the latter always starts from a single cell—the egg, which is the result of the fusion of two sexual cells, the gametes (a female–ovum, and a male – sperm). One of the reasons for intraindividual genetic heterogeneity is simply because in multicellular organisms dividing cells can accumulate copy errors (mutations) in their genetic makeup (BOX 1).

But the development of an egg can be troubled by many factors, and those reflected in the genetic material are of great interest in FG. From the FG point of view, it is useful to define two categories of accidents of development, including during adult life, which compromise the standard correspondence: one individual – one genome (and thus a single genetic profile).

The first category corresponds to the existence of two or more individuals with the same genome because they have resulted from a single egg: monozygotic twinning. Monozygotic ("single egged") twinning arises from the independent development of two embryos from the same egg. Therefore, these twins are of the same sex and unless copy errors occur during cell divisions (see below) their genetic makeup is the same.

Twinning, in the sense of the birth of two (or more) individuals at the same time, are not always due to the split of a single egg. Indeed, in the vast majority of cases, it results from the successful development of more than one egg. In this case, twins are said to be fraternal twins or dizygotic, literally meaning "two eggs". From the point of view of genetics, dizygotic twins are as different as siblings from different pregnancies (it may even occur that they have different fathers, so they are half-siblings). In some cases, the separation of the embryos (usually monozygotic) is not complete, giving rise to conjoined twins. This situation is easily identified, and therefore, poses no forensic problems.

The same happens with the fortunately rare twin-to-twin transfusion syndrome, in which twins share a placenta, and blood from one twin is diverted into the other twin. Since in the vast majority of the cases, the placenta sharing corresponds to monozygotic twinning, both have the same profile, forensically relevant implications are therefore rare.

In contrast, there are cases of 'hidden' dizygotic twinning, in which a single individual harbors a 'failed' sibling, having therefore a hybrid genetic makeup—a chimera (BOX 1). This situation can cause serious forensic errors, as the genetic profile of a certain part of the individual's body does not match the one obtained from a different body part. If chimerism involves the gamete forming parts of the body (BOX 1) and the individual's ovaries or testicles are involved, it may even cause a wrong kinship assignment. Indeed, as the biological sample used in these kinds of tests is usually blood or a buccal swab, the genetic profiles obtained from these fluids may not coincide with the ones that originated in the sperm or the ovum.

There is another sort of intraindividual heterogeneity that applies in particular to mtDNA (BOX 1), called heteroplasmy, which refers to the condition of possessing several types of mtDNA in the same individual. This condition is relatively frequent, due to their intrinsic high rate of mutation compared to nuclear DNA and to the high number of copies (hundreds to thousands) per cell.

FURTHER INFO

Castella, V., Lesta Mdel, M. and Mangin, P. (2009). One person with two DNA profiles: a(nother) case of mosaicism or chimerism. Int. J. Legal. Med., 123(5): 427–30. doi: 10.1007/s00414-009-0331-1.

Connell, J.R., Benton, M.C., Lea, R.A., Sutherland, H.G., Haupt, L.M. and Wright, K.M. (2022). Evaluating the suitability of current mitochondrial DNA interpretation guidelines for multigenerational whole mitochondrial genome comparisons. J. Forensic Sci., 00: 1–10. https://doi.org/10.1111/1556-4029.15097.

McElhoe, J.A., Wilton, P.R., Parson, W. and Holland, M.M. (2022). Exploring statistical weight estimates for mitochondrial DNA matches involving heteroplasmy. Int. J. Legal Med., 136(3): 671–685. doi: 10.1007/s00414-022-02774-5.

BOX 12

Investigating the Type of Biological Sample

Strictly speaking, the contribution of FG in court decisions is limited to the (sub)source level of propositions (↑ Introduction), that is to say, to provide quantified information on the individual who may have contributed to the sample. The court, however, is frequently interested in answering more complex, higher-level, alternative propositions. Namely, it may be relevant to elucidate which type of body fluid created a certain stain. This clarification may be important, for instance, in situations such as sexual assaults, in which both the level of criminal offense and the seriousness of the penalty are dependent, on the presence of either semen, vaginal secretions, blood (or menstrual blood), or saliva. For this, the contribution of FG exceeds the analysis of genetic material and its transmission and enters the realm of genetic expression. Thus, the detection of resulting products from the activity of genes or the distinctive modifications of the composition of the genetic material according to age (of the donor or the sample deposition), tissue of origin (skin, mucosa, etc.), or physiological status (menstrual blood, metabolic characteristics, etc.) may identify the origin of the stain.

The main difference between the practice of FG, in the strict sense (based on the genetic transmission theory), and these extensions is the difficulty—if not the impossibility—to frame the problems in terms of clear-cut alternative hypotheses and calculate probabilities (or expected frequencies) of the observations according to these premises. Therefore, explicitly or not, these FG extensions assume some sort of the discernable uniqueness principle. Even when solidly grounded on extensive empirical research data, results are not routinely (yet) reported in the form of likelihood ratios although some research on statistical methods has been developed for the prediction of the type of body fluid that could be the possible origin of a stain.

MORE INFO

de Zoete, J., Curran, J. and Sjerps, M. (2016). A probabilistic approach for the interpretation of RNA profiles as cell type evidence. Forensic Sci. Int. Genet., 20: 30–44. doi: 10.1016/j.fsigen.2015.09.007.

Dørum, G., Ingold, S., Hanson, E., Ballantyne, J., Snipen, L. and Haas, C. (2018). Predicting the origin of stains from next generation sequencing mRNA data. Forensic Sci. Int. Genet., 34: 37–48. doi: 10.1016/j.fsigen.2018.01.001.

Lindenbergh, A., Maaskant, P. and Sijen, T. (2013). Implementation of RNA profiling in forensic casework. Forensic Sci. Int. Genet., 7(1): 159–66. doi: 10.1016/j.fsigen.2012.09.003.

Varela Morillas, Á., Suhling, K. and Frascione, N. (2022). Unlocking the potential of forensic traces: Analytical approaches to generate investigative leads. Sci. Justice, 62(3): 310–326. doi: 10.1016/j.scijus.2022.03.005.

Watanabe, K., Taniguchi, K., Toyomane, K. and Akutsu, T. (2022). A new approach for forensic analysis of saliva-containing body fluid mixtures based on SNPs and methylation patterns of nearby CpGs. Forensic Sci. Int. Genet., 56: 102624. doi: 10.1016/j.fsigen.2021.102624.

Ypma, R.J.F., Maaskant-van Wijk, P.A., Gill, R., Sjerps, M. and van den Berge, M. (2021). Calculating LRs for presence of body fluids from mRNA assay data in mixtures. Forensic Sci. Int. Genet., 52: 102455. doi: 10.1016/j.fsigen.2020.102455.

BOX 13

Difficult Samples
Low Quantity/Quality;
Contamination & Mixtures

The most important technological advance in FG is doubtlessly resulting from the introduction of a method of amplifying selectively specific portions of the genetic material, DNA (↑Glossary). This technique (Polymerase Chain Reaction), usually known by the acronym PCR (↑Glossary), is basically a way of obtaining a great number of copies of the DNA present in a sample, which, as is typical in a forensic situation, may be vestigial and not sufficient for any analytical technique. PCR made therefore amenable to FG analyzes a wide range of traces that previously were useless for genotyping due to the very diminutive amount of DNA they contained, such as in stains or contacted surfaces (e.g., glass, cigarette buts, etc.).

As in any other technique, PCR, however, has limitations and risks of erroneous results. The first limitation is intrinsic to the technique: to start the amplification reaction, the addition of a pair of short pieces of DNA, known as primers, is required. These DNA sequences delimit the target DNA sample and therefore need to be complementary to its flanking region to obtain a successful PCR result. A previous study of the DNA genetic sequence of the organisms (human, for example, and/or other species) expected to have contributed to the sample is needed to determine the invariable stretches flanking the aimed variable genetic marker, where the primers will bind. Then, a failed amplification may result from the low quantity of undegraded DNA in the sample, but also from the lack of complementarity of the starters to the targeted DNA. Indeed, if the supposedly invariant sequence used for the primer design is altered in the analyzed individual, the complementation required for a reaction start is compromised and no reaction product is obtained. This failure, if total, does not imply reporting errors, since no genotype is assigned; however, since for most of the commonly used genetic markers, the genotype (↑Glossary) of an individual is dual, comprising two alleles (↑glossary), it can happen that just one of them will be missed, and the assigned genotype mistaken. The undetected allele thus behaves as a silent (↑Glossary) allele *s*, showing that, *even when applying DNA analysis, we have access to a phenotype* (↑Glossary) *and not the genotype*. This allele dropping is also prone to occur as a result of the low quantity of undegraded template DNA in the trace used as evidence; the chemical modifications occurring due to environmental insults or bad sample storage may furthermore be more frequent in some alleles leading to a systematic genotyping bias.

This is illustrated in the scheme below, in which the results of the analysis of an X-chromosome marker (DXS10101) in three female individuals (**a**, **b**, and **c**) are shown. It is clear that the genotype of **a** is 30–31, as two alleles are detected. In contrast, **b** and **c** both show a single peak, which means that their genotypes can be 30.2–30.2 or 30.2-*s*, and 28.2–28.2 or 28.2-*s*, respectively. In other words, both **b** and **c** can be either homozygous (↑glossary) or heterozygous (↑glossary)—carriers of a hidden silent allele, *s*. Therefore, when reporting, experts may only state the corresponding phenotypes: 30.2 and 28.2. Knowing that the height of the blue peaks is proportional to DNA quantity, we may nevertheless infer that, due to the low quantity of template DNA shown, the presence of the silent allele is more likely in the case of **c**, than in the case of **b**.

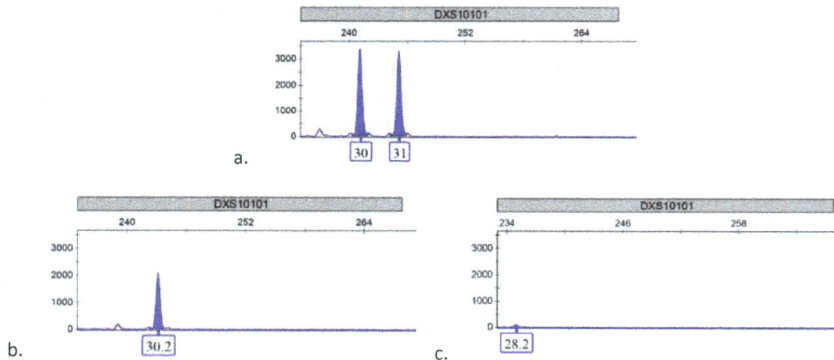

In fact, since PCR amplification is exponential, initial conditions are critical, and in the case of a starting DNA low copy number, it is possible, by mere chance, that one of the alleles present escapes the first rounds of amplification, leading to its total detection failure. A low quantity of template DNA can also produce other stochastic effects compromising the correct genotype inference, such as the amplification of spurious products (mistaken as true alleles). In conclusion, all PCR-based results —in particular those obtained from vestigial samples—must be interpreted with extreme care to avoid wrong conclusions.

The PCR's capacity of amplifying up to detectable levels minute amounts of DNA contained in a piece of evidence has also a dark side: it is especially vulnerable to contamination. Forensic samples at a crime scene are subject to many environmental insults and are easily contaminated in place, but also during collection and lab analysis, sometimes by the collectors or analysts themselves. The rigorous observation of a documented, unbroken chain of custody is therefore essential.

In consequence, it is not surprising that outside the scope of controlled collection of reference samples, a great proportion of the results of FG analyses reveals the presence of more than one contributor. These samples are characterized as mixtures and are typically those recovered from crime scenes, for example.

In these cases, more than two alleles are observed for some of the markers, which implies the existence of more than two contributors, as depicted below.

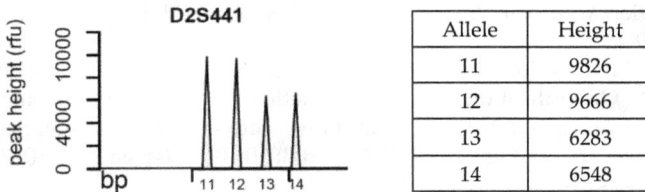

Allele	Height
11	9826
12	9666
13	6283
14	6548

The number of contributors to a mixture cannot be inferred, as well as the individual genetic profile of such donors. Anyway, the four peaked profile shown allows to infer that at least two donors contributed to the sample. A list of pairwise genotypic configurations is compatible with such a mixture (even assuming the minimum as the true number of contributors): 11–12 and 13–14; 11–13 and 12–14; 11–14 and 12–13. Again, under the assumption of two contributors, individual genotypes can be probabilistically inferred when using the relative peak heights of the alleles (taken as proxy of DNA quantity) information. This analysis may be carried out directly by the FG expert or using a dedicated software tool. In the case above, two peak pairs have quite distinct heights: one around 9,700 and the other ~ 6,400 which suggests (again assuming just two contributors) that individuals with genotypes 11–12 and 13–14 have contributed to the mixture. Nevertheless, with higher or lower likelihood (depending on the allele frequencies involved and the number of contributors), many other possibilities do exist and must be evaluated. In the case of autosomal markers, where independence between loci is likely, the obtaining of a complete individual profile is still not possible even when genotypes for some markers are estimated. The interpretation of these results is most of the times difficult, very prone to confirmation biases, and is far from consensual among the scientific community.

FURTHER INFO

Addendum to "SWGDAM Interpretation Guidelines for Autosomal STR Typing by Forensic DNA Testing Laboratories" to Address Next Generation Sequencing. https://www.swgdam.org/_files/ugd/4344b0_91f2b89538844575a9f51867def7be85.pdf.

Butler, J. (2014). Advanced Topics in Forensic DNA Typing: Interpretation. Elsevier Academic Press, San Diego, CA. https://doi.org/10.1016/C2011-0-07649-4.

Costa, C., Figueiredo, C., Amorim, A., Costa, S., Ferreira, P.M. and Pinto, N. (2022). Quantification of forensic genetic evidence: Comparison of results obtained by qualitative and quantitative software for real casework samples. Forensic Sci. Int. Genet., 59: 102715. doi: 10.1016/j.fsigen.2022.102715.

BOX 14

Probabilities, Likelihoods, and Ratios

The common notion of probability, usually known as the frequentist concept, is based on the previous knowledge of the occurrence of an event over a certain time period. More generally, it is also applied to the extrapolation of the proportion of a certain class of objects among a sampled collection. That is the meaning usually employed in genetics when we speak about the probability of an allele or a genotype: having sampled a population, and typing the individuals for a certain genetic marker, say the Rh blood group, we observe that 20% are negative (and 80% positive). From this experience, we therefore expect that any random individual from that population will be Rh negative with a probability of 20%.

The same information can also be conveyed in the form of an odds ratio, in which we say, for instance that the odds in favor of a random individual of that population being Rh positive is 80 against 20, or 4:1.

In a forensic genetics case, the value of the evidence is quantified through the computation of a likelihood ratio (LR). Such LR allows the comparison between the probabilities of the genetic observations, O, assuming alternative hypotheses, H_1 and H_2:

$$LR = \frac{P(O \mid H_1)}{P(O \mid H_2)}$$

This measure itself may be apparently difficult to interpret, as the quantification of interest would rely on the posterior odds (PO), obtained through the comparison of the probabilities of the alternative hypotheses, H1 and H2, given the genetic observations O:

$$PO = \frac{P(H_1 \mid O)}{P(H_2 \mid O)}$$

These two measures are however linked by the Bayes' theorem as follows:

$$PO = \frac{P(H_1)}{P(H_2)} \times LR$$

The ratio $P(H_1)/P(H_2)$ represents the prior odds and concerns the relative prior probabilities of the hypotheses before the genetic data is known. It is noteworthy that the establishment of the prior odds is outside the scope of geneticist's responsibility, being typically established by the court or the jurors. Prior odds are established considering any other sources of evidence beyond the genetics and may change during the legal process as more evidence become available. Given the subjectivity adjacent the prior odds (which quantification may vary from jurors to jurors), in most cases, the hypotheses at stake are considered *a priori* equally likely, which lead that PO and LR coincide. Indeed, the LR is the only objective quantification of the evidence to be presented in the court.

Such as the prior odds, hypotheses H_1 and H_2, must be carefully established independently and, ideally, before any knowledge on the genetic data. These hypotheses were usually referred as H_p and H_d, hypotheses of prosecution and defense, respectively, but these terms are slowly falling into disuse.

For example, in an identification case where the genetic profile of a suspect (person of interest, POI) needs to be compared with the one of a mixture sample recovered from crime scene, hypotheses H_1 and H_2 are typically established as:

H_1: DNA originated from the person of interest (POI) and N-1 unknown, unrelated individual(s), and H_2: DNA originated from N unknown, unrelated, individuals, where N represents the estimated number of contributors.

Similarly, in a standard paternity test involving a duo: alleged father (AF)/child (C), hypotheses are typically established as:

H_1: The individuals AF and C are related as parent-child, and

H_2: The individuals AF and C are unrelated.

At this point it should be emphasized that these hypotheses must be mutually exclusive and fully descriptive of the possible kin links existing between the individuals or samples. For example, if the alleged father may be a sibling of the real one, this should be clearly hypothesized as it will influence the calculations. The same occurs, for example, in an incest situation where the alleged father is related with the mother of the child.

When independent markers are used, as is generally the case for those included in commercial kits, this LR calculation is computed for each marker and the final result is obtained multiplying all the LRs obtained for each marker. Specifically for identification and paternity problems, this LR value may reach extremely high values. For example, if in a paternity test the LR obtained for each marker equals 2, that is, the probability of the observation is two times greater assuming the paternity than the alternative hypothesis, after analyzing 15 independent markers the LR amounts to 32,768.

MORE INFO

Caliebe, A. and Krawczak, M. (2016). Probability and likelihood. pp. 61–78. *In*: Amorim, A. and Budowle, B. (eds.). Handbook of Forensic Genetics. World Scientific Publishing Europe, London. https://doi.org/10.1142/9781786340788_0004.
Morrison, G.S. (2022). Advancing a paradigm shift in evaluation of forensic evidence: The rise of forensic data science, Forensic Science International: Synergy, 100270, https://doi.org/10.1016/j.fsisyn.2022.100270.
Swofford, S. and Champod, C. (2022). Probabilistic reporting and algorithms in forensic science: Stakeholder perspectives within the American criminal justice system. Forensic Science International: Synergy, 4: 100220, https://doi.org/10.1016/j.fsisyn.2022.100220.
Taroni, F., Garbolino, P., Bozza, S. and Aitken, C. (2021). The Bayes' factor: The coherent measure for hypothesis confirmation. Law, Probability and Risk, 20(1): 15–36, https://doi.org/10.1093/lpr/mgab007.

BOX 15

DNA Databases

Human forensic DNA databases (HFDNAD) are (at present) repositories of identified genetic profiles (↑Glossary), and/or unidentified profiles obtained from crime scene samples. These databases have widely different regulations from country to country, a fact that has a profound impact on their diverse efficiency for combating crime at the national and international levels. In some cases, they may also include samples relevant for missing persons' identification, not necessarily involving a crime.

One of these regulatory differences concerns the *inclusion criteria* for insertion of identified profiles in the databases. Indeed, no country has implemented a universal HFDNAD, and some possess very restrictive laws (such as limiting the inclusion to convicted offenders of serious crimes), while others, on the contrary, allow inclusively the insertion of mere suspects. There is also a great diversity of criteria for the *admissibility of unidentified profiles* obtained from crime samples, from those admitting mixture profiles (i.e., in which the contribution of more than one individual is acknowledged) to those only allowing the insertion of 'clean' profiles (i.e., which can be interpreted as having origin in a single individual).

Another aspect is the composition of the genetic profiles in terms of *genetic markers* (↑Glossary). When HFDNADs started (the first, UK-based, in 1995) the number of genetic markers was very small and had, therefore, a limited informative power, leading to a non-negligible rate of false matches (i.e., the probability of finding two different individuals with the same profile). The situation improved substantially and, at least for most national HFDNADs, this chance is, in practical terms, virtually impossible. However, there subsists a lack of uniformity of the adopted markers across countries, the consequence of it being that in some cases for which transnational queries are used, the number of overlapping markers is reduced, decreasing therefore the informative power, and increasing the risk of erroneous matches.

Besides the number, the nature of the genetic markers also deserves a close attention. It was consensual in the initial times of the HFDNADs that permissible markers should not reveal any physical characteristic of the individual, namely those related to health status or predispositions. This unanimity seems to be breaking apart, raising serious ethical concerns. Classically, HFDNADs included only non-sex-linked, biparentally transmitted genetic markers, so that this transmission mode (↑Glossary) was implicitly assumed when referring to "genetic markers". Meanwhile, it became popular and technically feasible to use other type of markers, namely those of uniparental transmission, common to either maternal (mtDNA ↑BOX 5) or paternal (Y chromosome ↑BOX 5) lineages. In consequence, some countries began introducing Y chromosome and mtDNA data, although with limitations, such as being used only in missing persons investigations. Again, this use is not exempt of ethically based criticisms, some of which is related to another facet of the heterogeneity of the HFDNADs, the question of what queries are allowed to perform. At this point, it should be remarked that both Y chromosome and mtDNA are lineage markers (paternal and maternal, respectively), which means that the analysis of these markers implies that not only the individuals or donors listed in the HFDNADs themselves, but also their paternal and maternal relatives, respectively, as well. Indeed, if the biparental markers may provide insights on the relatives of the individuals listed in the HFDNADs as we will see later, the situation of uniparental ones is even more sensitive.

The typical baseline of the HFDNADs use is the search for a match between a stored, identified profile and one found in a sample collected at crime scene, which can then be used as evidence against a suspect. The fact that most HFDNADs also contain unidentified profiles from ongoing or closed investigations allows the occurrence of a match between those unidentified profiles associated with distinct crimes. Therefore, this match, although not resulting in an immediate identification, by connecting to the same offender crimes thought to be unrelated, can provide an investigation lead based on their common circumstances. That is the case, for example, when the genetic profile recovered from various house burglaries, despite their wide geographic dispersion, is the same.

Otherwise, when no exact match is observed, there are often *partial matches* found, that is, two or more profiles (a) do match for all genetic markers, except for a few (say, one or two out of more than 15), or (b) they share at least one allele (↑Glossary) in all markers analyzed. This partial match can be interpreted as resulting from close genetic relationship between the donors of the partially matching profiles (BOX 7). Again, this can provide a substantial narrowing of the set of suspects leading the investigation to concentrate on the close relatives of the identified profile stored. When performed systematically this procedure — also hotly debated on ethical grounds— is called *familial searching* and although currently allowed in a few countries, is unregulated or forbidden in many others.

Transnational cooperation in using HFDNADs also faces difficulties not only because of the heterogeneity in the genetic markers employed, as explained above, but also by the profound differences at the regulatory level, namely on what information can be provided in the answer to a cross-border query.

Concerning *non-human DNA databases*, despite the growing need for individual identification, such as in cases of attacks on humans by a suspected dog, there is not yet available a resource similar to the standard HFDNADs. Forensic laboratories dealing with non-human material are forced to either produce in-house databases or rely on databases that were not built for forensic usage and are therefore of limited value for its application in this field.

FURTHER INFO

Machado, H., Granja, R. and Amorim, A. (2022). Ethical challenges of merging criminal identification and civil identification within the Prüm system. Forensic Sci. Int. Genet., 57: 102660. doi: 10.1016/j.fsigen.2022.102660.

Quinton, A.R., Kelty, S.F. and Scudder, N. (2022). Attitudes towards police use of consumer/private DNA databases in investigations. Sci. Justice., 62(3): 263–271. doi: 10.1016/j.scijus.2022.02.009.

Wickenheiser, R.A. (2022). Expanding DNA database effectiveness. Forensic Science International: Synergy, 4: 100226, https://doi.org/10.1016/j.fsisyn.2022.100226.

BOX 16

Combining Evidence from Different Genetic Markers

Most of the data used to calculate the probatory value of the evidence results from the analysis of standard genetic markers (↑Glossary) with a biparental mode of transmission (BOX 5). In this situation, provided that the markers used are not associated in some form and are independently transmitted to the offspring (BOX 8), the likelihood of the evidence obtained from the different markers can be combined in a simple, multiplicative fashion (BOX 14). This is generally the case when biparental markers are analyzed.

There are, however, many forensically relevant situations in which the typing of biparental markers proves to be difficult, due to a variety of technical limitations (BOX 13), and when the amount of information they provide is considered insufficient (BOX 7). Then, it may be helpful to analyze other markers, such as those from mtDNA or Y chromosome which have been widely used since the last century, and, more recently, from the X chromosome (BOX 5).

The problems arising from the usage of mtDNA and Y chromosome markers are of an ethical nature (BOX 18) but also computational and statistical, and directly result from their specific uniparental mode of transmission. Indeed, being uniparentally transmitted, these markers identify either maternal or paternal lineages and are thus unable to contribute to positive individual identification. This limitation is easily demonstrated with the example of the Y chromosome, which is exclusively transmitted from fathers to sons. In fact, barring mutations (↑Glossary), all members of a male lineage will share the same Y profile. In consequence, when observing a match between the suspect's Y-chromosome genetic profile and the one found in a crime scene sample, it is impossible to rule out a potentially great number of male relatives of the suspect (or of the crime scene donor). Nevertheless, despite being unable to provide positive individual identification, lineage markers are very effective for exclusion. Conversely, closely related individuals may not share the Y chromosomal profiles. For example, two maternal half-brothers are not expected to share the Y chromosomal profile, the probability of such occurrence being the same as for unrelated males.

Some experts, however, propose the combination of the likelihood ratios (BOX 14) obtained from uniparental markers with those from standard, biparental, ones into a single likelihood ratio. Their argument is on the basis that is feasible at least in some cases, to exclude, using other non-genetic types of information, the involvement of all relatives except the suspect. We do believe, however, that this possibility is quite remote, and easily questioned by the defense. Notwithstanding, from our point of view, the main objection to this proposal is strictly logico-mathematical — it is simply erroneous to combine likelihood ratios that were formulated according to different hypotheses. Indeed, while in the case of biparental markers and identification problems, the hypothesis is individual (and thus the probability of the observation under the hypothesis corresponds to the expected frequency of the individual genetic type), in the case of uniparental transmission, the hypothesis is collective (and the probability of the observation under the hypothesis is the frequency of a genetic lineage).

Note that we are not opposing the use, in the same case, of genetic evidence obtained from different types of markers. We simply consider it incorrect to report the results via a single likelihood ratio. The court is obviously free to use any form of combination of the genetic evidence delivered in the report, provided their different natures are understood. For that, a final cautionary remark is required. In practical terms, the recruitment of other markers besides the standard biparental is done when the evidence provided by them is deemed insufficient. This insufficiency can be due to two types of causes: typing technical difficulties (BOX 13) or unknown kinship between the suspect and the individual truly involved in the case. It is therefore risky, to say the least, to use inconsiderately information which biases the decision towards the wrong inclusion of a relative.

FURTHER INFO

Amorim, A. (2008). A cautionary note on the evaluation of genetic evidence from uniparentally transmitted markers. Forensic Science International: Genetics, 2: 376–378. doi: 10.1016/j.fsigen.2008.04.001.

Buckleton, J.S., Krawczak, M. and Weir, B.S. (2011). The interpretation of lineage markers in forensic DNA testing. Forensic Sci. Int. Genet., 5(2): 78–83. doi: 10.1016/j.fsigen.2011.01.010.

BOX 17

Exclusions

"Exclusion" is a word that corresponds to various concepts and situations, sometimes ill-defined and therefore so prone to confusions and misunderstandings leading to serious errors, that its usage in FG would best be avoided. Unfortunately, due to its apparent intuitiveness, it remains dangerously popular and therefore a careful analysis of the concepts behind it is mandatory.

Exclusion of what or whom?

The word is quite frequently used in the context of kinship investigations, mostly in paternity, in statements like "the alleged father PF is excluded" or "PF is excluded from being the father of C". It is considered in these statements that, given the observed genetic results, the biological kinship is impossible. What kind of genetic results are used to justify this categorical conclusion? Those in which the observed genetic profiles show an (apparent) contradiction between the claimed kinship and the assumed genetic transmission rules of (one or more) of the genetic markers (↑Glossary). When such an (apparent) contradiction is observed, it is commonly labeled as an "exclusion".

113

It is clear that these observations reveal in fact an *incompatibility*, which indeed, *may be due* to falsely alleged kinship, but may equally well result from *the inadequacy of the assumed genetic model*. Therefore, there is absolutely no basis for the biased interpretation of the results as a categorical kinship exclusion. Indeed, the incongruent results can be reconciled with the biological relationship, acknowledging that the problem may result from the model inadequacy. In practical terms, this situation is particularly relevant when very few incompatibilities are found, as we will explain later.

We will detail this in the framework of a paternity problem, focusing on a genetic marker in which the incompatibility is found, assuming a codominant (↑Glossary), non-sex-linked mode of transmission. Suppose we observe that the putative father PF is typed as 15 and the child C as 20. Assuming codominance, the results are interpreted as corresponding to the genotypes (↑Glossary) 15–15 and 20–20. However, most of the routine typing techniques are, in fact, unable to provide this information, so an unbiased analysis would also consider the possibility of the presence of a silent allele *s* (↑Glossary) and the corresponding genotypes would be, respectively, 15-*s* and 20-*s*, which, needless to say, are fully compatible with the biological paternity. Silent alleles are not quite common, and the estimation of their frequency is difficult (↑BOX 9), but in practice, a detection limit of 0.5% is acceptable. We are now able, instead of the categorical conclusion, to calculate, as generally recommended (Chapter I. Introduction/Quantification the probatory value of the evidence) a likelihood ratio (↑Glossary) — see BOX 14.

The hypotheses at stake are

H1: PF is the biological father of C

H2: PF is genetically unrelated to C

and then the expected frequency of the results will be

P(R|H1): The expected frequency of the results assuming H1

(a true father/child type 15-*s*/20-*s*); and

P(R|H2): The expected frequency of the results assuming H2

(a pair of unrelated individuals 15 (either 15–15 or 15-s)/20 (either 20–20 or 15-s),

allowing to compute the **ratio**:

$$LR = \frac{P(R|H1)}{P(R|H2)}$$

Depending on the frequency of the alleles (20 and the silent *s*), R can be either smaller or greater than 1, implying that *an apparent "exclusion" can instead constitute evidence in favor of paternity.*

Not all genetic incompatibilities between father and child can however be solved by invoking a silent allele. Suppose we observe, again assuming a codominant, non-sex-linked mode of transmission, that the putative father PF is typed as 15–16 and child 14–17. Once more, the erroneous categorical exclusionary conclusion of paternity seems obvious, but to do so we need to biasedly forget the possibility of mutation (↑Glossary). That makes us able to compute, as before, a likelihood ratio (↑Glossary)—see BOX 14. The hypotheses at stake are the same:

H1: PF is the biological father of C

H2: PF is genetically unrelated to C

and the conditional frequencies will now be

P(R|H1): The expected frequency of the results assuming H1

(a true father/child type 15–16/14–17, with mutation); and

P(R|H2): The expected frequency of the results assuming H2

(a pair of unrelated individuals 15–16/14–17)

allowing the computation of the **ratio**:

$$LR = \frac{P(R|H1)}{P(R|H2)}$$

Note that although individually rare (for the genetic markers currently used in commercial kits of the order of 1/1000), various mutations can occur in this specific case, reconciling the observations (PF: 15–16, and C: 14–17) with true biological paternity (for instance, 15 mutating to 14 or 16 to 17, just to mention the most frequent). Therefore, again this *"exclusion" can simply constitute quantitative evidence against paternity,* which is obviously quite different from excluding it. Compared with the situation where the incompatibility is explainable by the presence of a silent allele, in this case the LR is always smaller than 1, favoring (albeit sometimes weakly) the hypothesis of unrelatedness.

How many incompatibilities for an "exclusion"?

Real forensic paternity cases are quite frequently exempt from incompatibilities not only because events leading to incompatibilities are rare (both silent alleles and mutations) but also because in most situations, the real biological father is presented (not so when challenging established paternity), which biases the sampling towards the situations in which the questioned kinship is true. The FG expert is obviously prevented to apply this unquantified knowledge to the specific case under discussion.

There is a persistent tendency to suggest or recommend 'rules of the thumb' using the number of observed incompatibilities to establish a threshold legitimating a categorical exclusionary conclusion. From the above discussion, it must have clearly resulted that the only unbiased way to deal with the not so infrequent situation of observing (one or more instances of) incompatibility is to report the data in a uniform quantitative way, considering the possible occurrence of either silent alleles or mutations, irrespective of the presence among the genetic markers of one or more "exclusions". However, proposals go on being made, advocating the report of the qualitative dichotomy 'excluded/non-excluded' when the number of exclusionary markers exceeds a certain threshold (usually two or three). These proposals are unacceptable since 'exclusions' are frequently weak evidence against paternity and on some occasions, even in favor of it (when dealing with rare alleles), and its chance of occurrence must be properly quantified.

In conclusion, the use of the 'exclusion' approach, shown to be biased and formally incorrect, must be abandoned, and a uniform quantification of the evidence is mandatory. Moreover, publicly available software exists able to integrate both types of phenomena (silent alleles and mutations) which can lead to 'exclusions' between biologically related individuals into the calculation of a global likelihood ratio.

FURTHER INFO

Familias: Book, R version and Courses. https://familias.
    name/?msclkid=3eb28eb2d08911ecb16facc1a1e637f2.

BOX 18

The Life Network & Viruses

The commonly accepted view of the current diversity of organisms on the planet posits that all existing organisms are genealogically related in the more or less distant past and considers a single origin of life and the existence of a common ancestor, LUCA, an acronym for last universal common ancestor.

This view entails that all extant organisms are genetically connected: two (human) sibs at a truly short range, while for a human and a chimpanzee, the most recent common ancestor (MRCA) lived a few (~ 6) million years ago. The MRCA of all animals existed well before 500 million years ago and the origin of life began around 4,000 million years back.

The existence of LUCA does not mean that other events giving rise to different forms of life have not occurred, but simply that if they happened, no descendants were left (or were not found yet). This general picture is consistent with the observations (both from the genetic analyses and the fossil record), agreeing that the genetic relationship between all organisms allows their representation as a global genealogical tree (the Tree of Life, ToL). It does not imply that all genetic information present in an organism is transmitted vertically, as a genealogical tree suggests; in fact, a part of the genome (↑Glossary) of virtually all organisms has been the result of horizontal gene transfer (HGT), the incorporation of pieces of genetic material from organisms other than their ancestors. HGT is particularly frequent among unicellular (BOX 1) organisms but is far from exclusive to them: humans too, have parts of the genome that are explained as resulting from HGT.

HGT can result from various biological processes, but one that requires special attention is mediated by viruses. Viruses cannot be considered as living organisms, as they lack the ability to reproduce independently, depending on true living beings to replicate. The processes used by viruses to genetically parasitize a host are diverse, but in some of them they can (a) incorporate genetic material from the host into their own, and then transmit it to other organisms they can subsequently infect, as well as (b) have their genetic material permanently incorporated into the host's genome. Some of these insertions are far from detrimental to the host, and for instance, the mammalian reproduction seems to depend on a quite ancient one.

ToL morphology and topology (the branching and shape of the tree) are constantly being revised as new data on genome sequences are accumulating. For our purpose, it is however sufficient to have a broad glimpse as shown in the next figure (from Wikipedia, 1860px-Phylogenetic_tree.svg.png (1860 × 1010) (wikimedia.org), consulted on 03/01/2022). Both Bacteria and Archaea are prokaryotes (BOX 1), simple, mostly unicellular microorganisms, while the Eukaryotes branch encompasses all organisms with nucleated cells, either uni- or multicellular. Note that the multicellular organisms that catch our daily attention, animals and plants (and fungi - yeasts, moulds, and mushrooms, a little less so) are packed together, meaning that their genetic distance is not as large as our anthropocentric view may suggest. On the contrary, the branches of the humble, microscopic Bacteria and Archaea span across most of the ToL, evidencing that the branch length tends to be roughly proportional to genetic distance. All branches coalesce in a trunk or root, the LUCA.

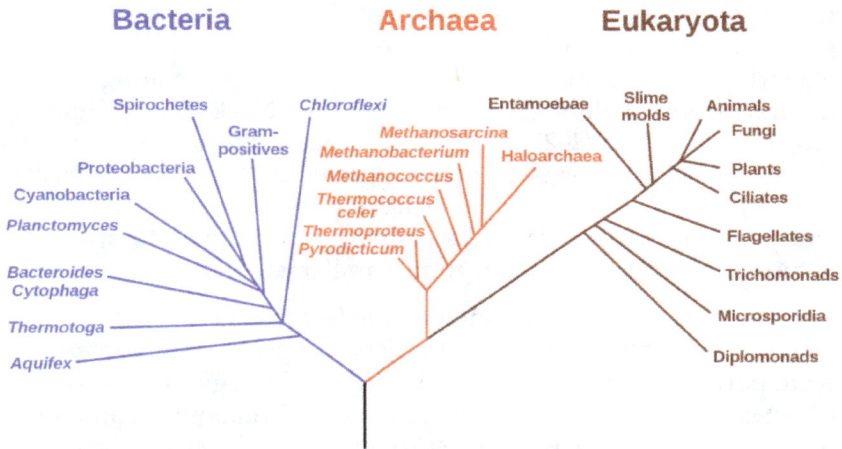

FURTHER INFO

Irwin, N.A.T., Pittis, A.A., Richards, T.A. and Keeling, P.J. (2021). Systematic evaluation of horizontal gene transfer between eukaryotes and viruses. Nat. Microbiol., 31. doi: 10.1038/s41564-021-01026-3.

Mayr, E. (1996). What is a Species, and What is Not? Philosophy of Science, 63(2): 262–277. doi:10.1086/289912.

Mi, S. et al. (2002). Syncytin is a captive retroviral envelope protein involved in human placental morphogenesis. Nature, 403: 785–789.

BOX 19

Genetically Modified Organisms (GMOs)

The legal definition of genetically modified organisms (GMOs) varies widely from country to country; the EU regulation, one of the most restrictive, states that a GMO is "an organism, with the exception of human beings, in which the genetic material has been altered in a way that does not occur naturally by mating and/or natural recombination" (EUR-Lex – l28130 – EN – EUR-Lex (europa. eu), consulted 28/12/2021). In any case, whatever the legal definition, the intention of the legislator (as suggested by the wording itself), is centered on the *process* originating the modified organism, irrespectively of the product resulting from the modification, focusing, explicitly or not, on "unnatural" methods.

These regulations were founded on the fear that new ("unnatural") technologies, able to change the genetic properties of an organism, were particularly risky and could produce damage to humans (by direct contact or consumption) or to the environment (by intended or inadvertent release of the GMOs). In consequence, any producer of a candidate GMO must subject it to extensive tests, before having its use authorized. It may therefore happen that the same GMO is authorized in some countries while being unauthorized in others. The forensic implications of this heterogeneity are obvious.

But, whatever the GMO definition (and the situation has recently gained a new facet with the introduction of the "bioengineered" label), either based on the process or the product (or both), the forensic verification of conformity to the pertinent law is laden with difficulties.

On the side of *detection of the process*, FG (or any other analytical approach) is limited by the available data on the methods employed in order to detect their signature in the materials to be examined.

However, most if not all relevant technical information required is usually kept confidential by the biotech company which developed the GMO, and even when this information is available, there is an obvious lack of harmonisation and standardisation of GMOs analysis. Moreover, entirely new methods are continuously being developed, and even some of the already existing ones leave no genomic 'scar' whatsoever to be detected. These include directed mutagenesis (↑Glossary) and various forms of gene editing (↑Glossary).

With regard to the *product detection*, it must be clarified that the GMO concept was developed at a time when the only genetic modification that could be thought of, was the stable insertion of a piece of genetic material from an organism on the genome (↑Glossary) of another one (the GMO). As seen above, many other modifications are now possible and are being applied that do not involve the incorporation of extraneous genetic material from another species. Therefore, quite often there is no 'abnormal' product to be detected since the genetic modification introduced just increases the level of expression of the desired gene (for instance, a growth factor).

FURTHER INFO

Chen, L., Zhou, J., Li, T., Fang, Z., Li, L., Huang, G., Gao, L., Zhu, X., Zhou, X., Xiao, H., Zhang, J., Xiong, Q., Zhang, J., Ma, A., Zhai, W., Zhang, W. and Peng, H. (2021). GmoDetector: An accurate and efficient GMO identification approach and its applications. Food Res. Int., 149: 110662. doi: 10.1016/j.foodres.2021.110662.

Henry Miller and Kathleen Hefferon. (2021). Is there a difference between a gene-edited organism and a 'GMO'? The question has important implications for regulation|Genetic Literacy Project May 12, 2021. https://geneticliteracyproject.org/2021/05/12/is-there-a-difference-between-a-gene-edited-organism-and-a-gmo-the-questin-has-important-implications-for-regulation/.

Moreira, F., Carneiro, J. and Pereira, F. (2017). A proposal for standardization of transgenic reference sequences used in food forensics. Forensic Science International Genetics, 29: e26-e28. DOI: 10.1016/j.fsigen.2017.04.022.

Steve Savage. (2022). Salmon, apples and potatoes — 3 healthy and sustainable foods that you can buy now under the new "bioengineered" label. I Genetic Literacy Project January 4, 2022. https://geneticliteracyproject. org/2022/01/04/viewpoint-salmon-apples-and-potatoes-3-healthy-and-sustainable-foods-that-you-can-buy-now-under-the-new-bioengineered-label/?mc_cid=fe0995cc72&mc_eid=8e8f0f296d.

Tagliabue, G. (2016). The meaningless pseudo-category of "GMOs": The trouble with the "new techniques" for genetically modifying crops demonstrates the illogical process-based definition of GMOs in EU regulation. EMBO Rep., 17(1): 10-3. doi: 10.15252/embr.201541385.

BOX 20

Ethical and Legal Issues

Although the realms of law and ethics are inextricably linked, the diversity of legislations and legal systems across countries prevent us from undertaking a useful analysis of the questions pertaining to the contents and the enforcement of legal procedures, dispositions, and regulations. As an illustrating and striking example, we mention the immense gap between the inquisitorial and adversarial systems in what deals with individual rights and the ways FG expertise is produced, admitted as evidence, by whom, and in what conditions it is admissible and subjectable to counterproof.

We will focus our attention on a few ethical aspects of the FG use, its processes, application, and practitioners' rules of conduct, which, despite significant changes in assumptions, beliefs, and perspectives in recent times, do have, nonetheless, a certain degree of universal acceptance.

Expert rules of conduct

It is widely accepted that forensic experts in general should be in a situation of *independence* relatively to conflicting parties. Unfortunately, most FG practitioners are employees (or work within the frame) of a law enforcement organization, such as police laboratories, or forensic institutes dependent of the nation's ministry of justice, or an equivalent governmental department. Needless to say, this situation seriously compromises the wished expert's independence, and not just on the grounds of his/her attitude and motivation. Indeed, it may even violate another assumed rule of conduct, that is, the *unbiased* production and evaluation of evidence. As an example, it is customary to analyze the genetic evidence from a crime scene with the knowledge of the genetic profile of the suspect. That knowledge inevitably leads to confirmation bias, which is especially serious in cases of vestigial samples and mixtures. In these conditions, the expert may tend to find the profile of the subject in a set of complex results prone to technical artifacts, for which alternative interpretations are possible.

Informed consent — individual and collective

The collection of biological samples from an individual is universally considered to require the donor's consent, whatever the purpose. It must be remarked that there is however a widely tolerated exception to this principle: the case of convicted offenders, or more generally, of persons fitting the inclusion criteria for contributing to a forensic DNA database (BOX 15).

It is also unanimously recognized that this consent is meaningless without the specification of the purpose of the sampling, which in our context is the obtention of the person's genetic data. Equally accepted is the concept that the donor should be informed of the nature of these data and their actual or potential uses; hence, an informed consent is mandatory. The concept, despite well-intentioned, is nevertheless difficult to apply to genetic data, which provides information about the donor's relatives, by their hereditary nature itself. That is particularly obvious for uniparentally transmitted markers (BOX 5), in which the individual consent directly discloses the corresponding information on all members of her/his paternal and/or maternal lineages. Although less directly, this disclosure happens with all genetic data whatever the transmission mode (BOXes 5–7), which undermines the idea behind the informed consent concept, that is, the ownership of one's genetic makeup.

The perception that our genetic information is indeed a shared heritage, has raised concerns at a population level, namely when minorities or small populations are studied. Although some proposals have been presented (such as the prerequisite of a poll to the community), no general solution has been advanced, but instances of paper retractions and removal of profiles from DNA databases on the grounds of doubtful ethical samplings have been recorded.

Familial searching: recreational and forensic databases

As explained above, a stored genetic profile is inherently a source of information, not only on the donor but also on his/her relatives. Being so, forensic DNA databases can be used to search for individual matches, but also family searches (BOX 15). The legal permission to perform such searches has raised many ethical criticisms, which have substantially grown when the so-called recreational genetic databases were used for police investigations. In this case, whatever contents have the informed consent of the participants, surely there was no mention of the possibility that they could serve police investigations and unwillingly incriminate an unconsented relative.

FURTHER INFO

Busey, T., Sudkamp, L., Taylor, M.K. and White, A. (2021). Stressors in forensic organizations: Risks and solutions, Forensic Science International: Synergy, 100198, https://doi.org/10.1016/j.fsisyn.2021.100198.

de Groot, N.F., van Beers, B.C. and Meynen, G. (2021). Commercial DNA tests and police investigations: A broad bioethical perspective. J. Med. Ethics, 47(12): 788–95. doi: 10.1136/medethics-2021-107568.

Hayden, E.C. (2012). Informed consent: A broken contract. Nature, 486(7403): 312–4. doi: 10.1038/486312a.

Hunter, P. (2021). Cold cases and ancient trade routes: DNA phenotyping and isotope analysis extend forensic science into new domains. EMBO Rep., 22(12): e54188. doi: 10.15252/embr.202154188.

Machado, H., Granja, R. and Amorim, A. (2022). Ethical challenges of merging criminal identification and civil identification within the Prüm system. Forensic Sci. Int. Genet., 57: 102660. doi: 10.1016/j.fsigen.2022.102660.

Mittelstadt, B.D. and Floridi, L. (2016). The ethics of Big Data: Current and foreseeable issues in biomedical contexts. Sci. Eng. Ethics, 22(2): 303-41. doi: 10.1007/s11948-015-9652-2.

Roffey, P. and Scudder, N. (2022). Privacy implications of the new "omic" technologies in law enforcement. WIREs Forensic Science, 4(3): e1445. https://doi.org/10.1002/wfs2.1445.

Samuel, G. and Prainsack, B. (2019). Civil society stakeholder views on forensic DNA phenotyping: Balancing risks and benefits. Forensic Sci. Int. Genet., 43: 102157. doi: 10.1016/j.fsigen.2019.102157.

Schiermeier, Q. (2021). Forensic database challenged over ethics of DNA holdings. Nature, 594(7863): 320–322. doi: 10.1038/d41586-021-01584-w. PMID: 34131337.

Syndercombe Court, D. (2018). Forensic genealogy: Some serious concerns. Forensic Sci. Int. Genet., 36: 203–204. doi: 10.1016/j.fsigen.2018.07.011.

Wickenheiser, R.A. (2019). Forensic genealogy, bioethics and the Golden State Killer case. Forensic Sci. Int. Synerg., 1: 114-125. doi: 10.1016/j.fsisyn.2019.07.003.

Wienroth, M., Granja, R., Lipphardt, V., Nsiah Amoako, E. and McCartney, C. (2021). Ethics as lived practice. anticipatory capacity and ethical decision-making in forensic genetics. Genes (Basel), 12(12): 1868. doi: 10.3390/genes12121868.

Williams, R. and Wienroth, M. (2017). Social and ethical aspects of forensic genetics: A critical review. Forensic Sci. Rev., 29(2): 145-169. PMID: 28691916.

Winburn, A.P. and Clemmons, C. (2021). Objectivity is a myth that harms the practice and diversity of forensic science. Forensic Science International Synergy, 3: 100196. https://doi.org/10.1016/j.fsisyn.2021.100196.

V
Annexes

Bibliographic and Web Resources

In this annex we provide a commented selected list of useful resources for those wanting to deepen the knowledge on forensic genetics. The first section comprises handbooks, the second topical and general reviews, while the last critically enumerates relevant sites and pages available on the Internet.

Textbooks

Amorim, A. and Budowle, B. (2016). Handbook of Forensic Genetics: Biodiversity and Heredity in Civil and Criminal Investigation. World Scientific, New Jersey. https://doi.org/10.1142/q0023.
Intends to bridge the barriers between legal medicine, biodiversity and conservation, and food analysis in an integrated forensic perspective.

Balding, D.J. and Steele, C.D. (2015). Weight-of-Evidence for Forensic DNA Profiles, 2nd ed. Wiley & Sons Ltd, ISBN: 978-1-118-81455-0
An advanced text on the statistical evaluation of evidence; developed chapters on population genetics and issues on the presentation of results in court and avoiding fallacies.

Bell, S. and Butler, J. (2022). Understanding Forensic DNA. Cambridge: Cambridge University Press. doi:10.1017/9781009043311 3.
Designed for a general readership; cases and examples discussed; probability calculation and dispelling common misunderstandings.

Bright, J.-A. and Coble, M. (2021). Forensic DNA Profiling: A Practical Guide to Assigning Likelihood Ratios. CRC Press. ISBN 9781032082318.
Designed for enabling the statistics underlying the formulation of likelihood ratios; introduces the required basis and proposition setting with special emphasis on mixtures.

Buckleton, J.S., Bright, J.-A. and Taylor, D. (2021). Forensic DNA Evidence Interpretation. 2nd ed. CRC Press. ISBN 9780367778101.
Claims to provide a link among the biological, forensic, and interpretative domains of the DNA profiling field and to be a resource for forensic scientists, technicians, molecular biologists, and attorneys; important presentation of subpopulation effects, and databases.

Butler, J.M. (2011). Advanced Topics in Forensic DNA Typing: Methodology. Academic Press. ISBN: 9780123745132.
Although aimed at forensic DNA analysts as its primary audience, includes a chapter on legal aspects of DNA testing to prepare scientists for expert witness testimony.

Cooper, J.E. and Cooper, M.E. (2013). Wildlife Forensic Investigation: Principles and Practice. CRC Press. ISBN 9780367778156.
Describes the application of forensic science (not just Genetics) to wildlife investigations and provides guidance to writing reports and appearing in court. Includes appendices on Standard Witness Statement and wildlife forensic cases (United Kingdom).

Erlich, H., Stover, E. and White, T.J. (2020). Silent Witness: Forensic DNA Evidence in Criminal Investigations and Humanitarian Disasters, New York, Oxford Academic Press. ISBN: 9780190909444.
Assuming that the scientific, legal and ethical concepts underlying DNA evidence remain unclear to the general public, judges, prosecutors, defense attorneys, and students of law, forensic sciences, ethics, and genetics it aims however at forensic practitioners as primary audience; and includes a chapter on legal aspects of DNA testing for expert witness testimony and another on microbial forensics.

Elkins, K.M. (2013). Forensic DNA Biology: A Laboratory Manual. Academic Press. https://doi.org/10.1016/C2011-0-06748-0.
Despite the subtitle, it contains a chapter on Social, Ethical, and Regulatory Concerns and another on Selected Forensic DNA Biology Case Studies.

Ferrero, A. and Scotti, V. (2022). Forensic Metrology. An Introduction to the Fundamentals of Metrology for Judges, Lawyers and Forensic Scientists. Research for Development. Springer, Cham. eBook ISBN 978-3-031-14619-0.
Presents the limits of validity of scientific evidence, discussing the fundamental concepts of metrology, and explains how metrology to quantify the reliability of measurement results. Includes informative case studies in which measurement of uncertainty has played and a full chapter on DNA profiling.

Goodwin, W. (2010). An Introduction to Forensic Genetics. John Wiley & Sons. 2nd ed. ISBN: 9780470010266.
Assumed to be an accessible introduction, includes the evaluation and presentation of DNA evidence in court and guidance on the evaluation process, suggesting how court reports and statements should be presented.

Huffman, J.E. and Wallace, J.R. (2012). Wildlife Forensics: Methods and Applications. Wiley. ISBN: 978-1-119-95314-2.
Although aimed to students and practitioners, it contains accessible analyses of cases of DNA application to wildlife forensics, including case studies and the specific difficulties of the field and quality control.

Jamieson, A. and Bader, S. (eds.). (2016). A Guide to Forensic DNA Profiling. John Wiley & Sons Ltd. ISBN: 978-1-118-75152-7.
A deep focus on analysis, interpretation, and evaluation of genetic evidence; embraces, among 'classical' applications, databases issues, wildlife, phenotyping inference, and familial searching; at court level, presents report writing, discovery, cross-examination, and current controversies.

Kobilinsky, L., Liotti, T.F. and Oeser-Sweat, J. (2004). DNA: Forensic and Legal Applications. Wiley. ISBN: 978-0-471-41478-0.
Despite the year of publication, contains still valuable analyses on the proceedings protocols during sample examination to results and on Legal Theory, namely on the admissibility of DNA evidence, attacking and defending DNA evidence, with human and non-human examples.

Lawless, C. (2022). Forensic Science: A Sociological Introduction. 2nd Edition. Routledge. ISBN 9780367647148.
Explores the integration of science into police work and criminal investigation, the relationship between law and science, and the ethical and social issues raised by new DNA analyses.

Linacre, A. (ed.). (2009). Forensic Science in Wildlife Investigations. CRC Press. ISBN 9780849304101.
Written at a level requiring a fundamental knowledge of biology; rather outdated.

131

Linacre, A. and Tobe, S. (2013). Wildlife DNA Analysis: Applications in Forensic Science. Wiley-Blackwell. ISBN: 978-0-470-66596-1.
Centered on forensic genetics of wildlife forensic science, addresses species testing and genetic kinship/identification/population assignment.

Machado, H. and Granja, R. (2020). Forensic Genetics in the Governance of Crime. Springer Nature. ISBN: 9789811524295.
A critical sociological perspective, examining the new challenges of the paradigm shift, from the construction of evidence to the production of intelligence guiding criminal investigations.

Morling, N. (ed.). (2022). Advances in Forensic Genetics. https://doi.org/10.3390/ books978-3-0365-4698-8.
A heterogeneous collection of articles published in a special issue of Genes; useful chapters on ethical issues, the value of genetic evidence from haploid markers (Y chromosome and mtDNA), DNA phenotyping (predicting visible traits), the logical framework for DNA interpretation, animal forensic genetics, the identification of body fluids and tissues, ancestry, and genealogy leads.

Semikhodskii, A. (2007). Dealing with DNA Evidence: A Legal Guide. Routledge-Cavendish. ISBN 9781845680497.
After a brief introduction to the interpretation and statistical evaluation of DNA evidence, examines interpretation errors and testing pitfalls and errors, discusses the challenging of DNA evidence in court and corresponding ethical aspects.

Taupin, J.M. (2013). Introduction to Forensic DNA Evidence for Criminal Justice Professionals. CRC Press. ISBN 9781439899090.
Designed for nonscientific readers on how to effectively use genetic evidence in criminal cases; developed analyses of concerns, misconceptions, and controversies, including advice for the prosecution and the defense, cross-examination questions and case examples, discovery requests and issues on the presentation of results in court avoiding fallacies.

Taupin, J.M. (2016). Using Forensic DNA Evidence at Trial: A Case Study Approach. CRC Press. ISBN 9781482255812.
Aimed for the non-scientific reader, presents a variety of cases, including familial searching and non-human examples, as well as a section on quality issues.

Williams, R. and Johnson, P. (2008). Genetic Policing: The Uses of DNA in Police Investigations. Routledge. ISBN 9781843922049.
Describes the relationship between scientific knowledge and police investigations and is illustrated by some of the major UK criminal cases in which DNA evidence has been presented and contested.

Reviews

Arenas, M., Pereira, F., Oliveira, M., Pinto, N., Lopes, A.M., Gomes, V., Carracedo, A. and Amorim, A. (2017). Forensic genetics and genomics: Much more than just a human affair. PLoS Genet., 13(9): e1006960. doi: 10.1371/journal. pgen.1006960.

Børsting, C. and Morling, N. (2015). Next generation sequencing and its applications in forensic genetics. Forensic Sci. Int. Genet., 18: 78–89. doi: 10.1016/j.fsigen.2015.02.002.

Butler, J.M. (2015). The future of forensic DNA analysis. Philos. Trans. R Soc. Lond. B Biol. Sci., 370(1674): 20140252. doi: 10.1098/rstb.2014.0252.

Collins, R.A. and Cruickshank, R.H. (2014). Known knowns, known unknowns, unknown unknowns and unknown knowns in DNA barcoding: A comment on Dowton et al. Syst. Biol., 63(6): 1005–9. doi: 10.1093/sysbio/syu060.

Dabas, P., Jain, S., Khajuria, H. and Nayak, B.P. (2022). Forensic DNA phenotyping: Inferring phenotypic traits from crime scene DNA. J. Forensic. Leg. Med., 88: 102351. doi: 10.1016/j.jflm.2022.102351.

Dash, H.R. and Arora, M. (2022). CRISPR-CasB technology in forensic DNA analysis: Challenges and solutions. Appl. Microbiol. Biotechnol., 106(12): 4367–4374. doi: 10.1007/s00253-022-12016-8.

de Knijff, P. (2019). From next generation sequencing to now generation sequencing in forensics. Forensic Sci. Int. Genet., 38: 175–180. doi: 10.1016/j. fsigen.2018.10.017.

Evett, I., Pope, S. and Puch-Solis, R. (2016). Providing scientific guidance on DNA to the judiciary. Science & justice: Journal of the Forensic Science Society, 56(4): 278–281. https://doi.org/10.1016/j.scijus.2016.05.001.

Foreman, L., Champod, C., Evett, I., Lambert, J. and Pope, S. (2003). Interpreting DNA evidence: A review. International Statistical Review, 71: 473–495. https://doi.org/10.1111/j.1751-5823.2003.tb00207.x.

Ge, J. and Budowle, B. (2021). Forensic investigation approaches of searching relatives in DNA databases. J. Forensic Sci., 66(2): 430–443. doi: 10.1111/1556-4029.14615.

Glynn, C.L. (2022). Bridging disciplines to form a new one: The emergence of forensic genetic genealogy. Genes (Basel)., 13(8): 1381. doi: 10.3390/genes13081381.

Gomes, I., Pinto, N., Antão-Sousa, S., Gomes, V., Gusmão, L. and Amorim, A. (2021). Twenty years later: A comprehensive review of the X chromosome use in forensic genetics. Front Genet., 11: 926. doi: 10.3389/fgene.2020.00926.

Ishak, S., Dormontt, E. and Young, J.M. (2021). Microbiomes in forensic botany: A review. Forensic Sci. Med. Pathol., 17(2): 297–307. doi: 10.1007/s12024-021-00362-4.

Iyengar, A. and Hadi, S. (2014). Use of non-human DNA analysis in forensic science: A mini review. Med. Sci. Law., 54(1): 41–50. doi: 10.1177/0025802413487522.

Jordan, D. and Mills, D. (2021). Past, present, and future of DNA typing for analyzing human and non-human forensic samples. Frontiers in Ecology and Evolution, 9. DOI=10.3389/fevo.2021.646130.

Just, R.S., Irwin, J.A. and Parson, W. (2015). Mitochondrial DNA heteroplasmy in the emerging field of massively parallel sequencing. Forensic Sci. Int. Genet., 18: 131–9. doi: 10.1016/j.fsigen.2015.05.003.

Kanthaswamy, S. (2015). Review: Domestic animal forensic genetics - biological evidence, genetic markers, analytical approaches and challenges. Anim. Genet., 46(5): 473–84. doi: 10.1111/age.12335.

Katsanis, S.H. (2020). Pedigrees and perpetrators: Uses of DNA and genealogy in forensic investigations. Annu. Rev. Genomics Hum. Genet., 21: 535–564. doi: 10.1146/annurev-genom-111819-084213.

Kayser, M. (2015). Forensic DNA phenotyping: Predicting human appearance from crime scene material for investigative purposes. Forensic Sci. Int. Genet., 18: 33–48. doi: 10.1016/j.fsigen.2015.02.003.

Kling, D., Phillips, C., Kennett, D. and Tillmar, A. (2021). Investigative genetic genealogy: Current methods, knowledge and practice. Forensic Sci. Int. Genet., 52: 102474. doi: 10.1016/j.fsigen.2021.102474.

Ogden, R. and Linacre, A. (2015). Wildlife forensic science: A review of genetic geographic origin assignment. Forensic Sci. Int. Genet., 18: 152–9. doi: 10.1016/j.fsigen.2015.02.008.

Oliveira, M. and Amorim, A. (2018). Microbial forensics: new breakthroughs and future prospects. Appl. Microbiol. Biotechnol., 102(24): 10377–10391. doi: 10.1007/s00253-018-9414-6.

Parson, W. (2018). Age estimation with DNA: From forensic DNA fingerprinting to forensic (Epi)Genomics: A mini-review. Gerontology, 64(4): 326–332. doi: 10.1159/000486239.

Smart, U., Cihlar, J.C. and Budowle, B. (2021). International Wildlife Trafficking: A perspective on the challenges and potential forensic genetics solutions. Forensic Sci. Int. Genet. doi: 10.1016/j.fsigen.2021.102551.

Taylor, D., Kokshoorn, B. and Biedermann, A. (2018). Evaluation of forensic genetics findings given activity level propositions: A review. Forensic Sci. Int. Genet., 36: 34-49. doi: 10.1016/j.fsigen.2018.06.001.

Tvedebrink, T. (2022). Review of the forensic applicability of biostatistical methods for inferring ancestry from autosomal genetic markers. Genes (Basel). doi: 10.3390/genes13010141.

Weir, B.S. (2019). Forensic genetics. *In*: Balding, D., Moltke, I., Marioni, J. (eds.). Handbook of Statistical Genomics. Wiley.https://doi.org/10.1002/9781119487845.ch18.

Williams, R. and Wienroth, M. (2017). Social and ethical aspects of forensic genetics: A critical review. Forensic Sci. Rev., 29(2): 145–169.

Web Resources

Journals

The only scientific journal entirely dedicated to Forensic Genetics is

Forensic Science International: Genetics
https://www.fsigenetics.com/

The Proceedings of the International Society for Forensic Genetics Congresses are published in the companion journal:

Forensic Science International: Genetics Supplement Series
https://www.sciencedirect.com/journal/forensic-science-international-genetics-supplement-series

Some other, broader journals do publish relevant articles, such as

Journal of Forensic Sciences
https://www.aafs.org/journal-forensic-sciences, the official publication of the American Academy of Forensic Sciences

Forensic Science International
https://www.sciencedirect.com/journal/forensic-science-international

Forensic Science International: Animals and Environments
https://www.sciencedirect.com/journal/forensic-science-international-animals-and-environments

Forensic Science International: Reports
https://www.sciencedirect.com/journal/forensic-science-international-reports

Forensic Science International: Synergy
https://www.sciencedirect.com/journal/forensic-science-international-synergy

Environmental Forensics
https://www.tandfonline.com/journals/uenf20, the official journal of the International Society of Environmental Forensics

Science & Justice
https://www.journals.elsevier.com/science-and-justice, the official journal of The Chartered Society of Forensic Sciences

The American Journal of Forensic Medicine and Pathology
https://journals.lww.com/amjforensicmedicine/Pages/aboutthejournal.aspx

Journal of Forensic and Legal Medicine
https://journals.elsevier.com/journal-of-forensic-and-legal-medicine

International Journal of Legal Medicine
https://www.springer.com/journal/414

Forensic Sciences Research
https://www.tandfonline.com/journals/tfsr20

Scientific Societies and Networks

American Academy of Forensic Sciences https://www.aafs.org/
Asian Forensic Sciences Network https://asianforensic.net/
Association of Forensic DNA Analysts and Administrators https://afdaa.org/2021/
European Forensic Genetics Network of Excellence EUROFORGEN https://www.euroforgen.eu/
European Network of Forensic Science Institutes https://enfsi.eu/
Forensic Expert Witness Association https://forensic.org/
Innocence Project - Expanding Knowledge https://innocenceproject.org/Educate/
Interpol | Wildlife crime | Environmental crime https://www.interpol.int/Crimes/Environmental-crime/Wildlife-crime
International Society for Animal Genetics https://www.isag.us/index.asp
International Society for Forensic Genetics https://www.isfg.org/
International Society of Environmental Forensics http://www.environmentalforensics.org/
Society for Wildlife Forensic Science https://www.wildlifeforensicscience.org/
The British Academy of Forensic Sciences https://www.bafs.org.uk/index.php
The Chartered Society of Forensic Sciences https://www.csofs.org/
The International Consortium on Combating Wildlife Crime | CITES https://cites.org/eng/prog/iccwc_new.php
The Organization of Scientific Area Committees for Forensic Science (OSAC) https://www.nist.gov/organization-scientific-area-committees-forensic-science
United Nations Office on Drugs and Crime (unodc.org) https://www.unodc.org/unodc/index.html;
World Wildlife Report (unodc.org)
Wildlife Forensic Science http://www.wildlifeforensicscience.org/

Databases

EMPOP - mtDNA database https://empop.online/
STRBase - https://strbase.nist.gov/index.htm

STRidER - STRs for identity ENFSI Reference database https://strider.online/
YHRD - Y Chromosome Haplotype Reference Database https://yhrd.org/

Forensically Involved Companies

Applied Biosystems ⏐ Thermo Fisher Scientific – https://www.thermofisher.com/
   pt/en/home/brands/applied-biosystems.html
Promega Corporation - https://worldwide.promega.com/; Resources (promega.
   com)
QIAGEN - https://www.qiagen.com/us/applications/human-identity-and-forensics
Thermo Fisher Scientific - https://www.thermofisher.com/pt/en/home/industrial/
   forensics.html

Annotated Mock Reports

In this annex, we provide a few examples of mock reports corresponding to some of the Q&As of the main text, commented and annotated, and highlighting the assumptions used and their possible violation. Some are modified from

Amorim, A., Crespillo, M., Luque, J.A., Prieto, L., Garcia, O., Gusmão, L., Aler, M., Barrio, P.A., Saragoni, V.G. and Pinto, N. (2016). Formulation and communication of evaluative forensic science expert opinion — A GHEP-ISFG contribution to the establishment of standards. Forensic Sci. Int. Genet., 25: 210–213. doi: 10.1016/j.fsigen.2016.09.003.

The internal forms mentioned in the reports concern laboratory specific documentation that will not be shown as they differ from laboratory to laboratory.

Mock reports for the following problems will be presented:
  I. Mock report for a case of identification
 II. Mock reports for paternity cases
     a. Standard putative father/child duo: Paternity not excluded
     b. Standard putative father/mother-child trio: Paternity practically excluded
     c. Complex putative father/child duo: Putative father possibly related to the real one
     d. Complex putative father/mother-child trio: The putative father related to the mother of the child

III. Mock reports for complex kinship cases

    a. Sibship problem

    b. Incest problem: Alleged and absent father related to the mother of the child

IV. Mock report for a case of species identification

I. Mock report for a case of identification

This case corresponds to the Q&A 01:

Human identification: Is this trace from John Doe?

These problems concern situations where the aim is, generally speaking, to evaluate the likelihood of an identified individual having contributed to an unidentified sample. This is the typical case in a criminal context, where, for example, a reference sample recovered from a suspect is compared with a stain recovered from a crime scene.

Comparison of genetic profiles between trace and suspect

Although formally identical, the example report is presented in a non-criminal context, assuming a genuine, uncontaminated (has a single source) trace, present in sufficient amount and reasonable preservation conditions. In the exemplified situation, there was a suspicion that a diagnosis (and subsequent treatment) was based on a swapped sample. Further information on the case can be found at: Alonso, A. et al. (2005). Mitochondrial DNA haplotyping revealed the presence of mixed up benign and neoplastic tissue sections from two individuals on the same prostatic biopsy slide. J. Clin. Pathol., 58(1): 83–6. DOI: 10.1136/jcp.2004.017673.

For simplicity's sake this report is presented considering qualitative conclusions regarding single source samples. However, a quantification of the observations, as obtained in the reports II.a. to II.d., III.a. and III.b., could also be obtained resorting to appropriate software in complex situations involving samples from more than one contributor.

Report I

Identity Test n° xxx/yyyy

XXX requested the comparison of the genetic profiles between

- the reference sample from *XXX* and the biological material from a slide biopsy, coded SB1;
- the reference sample from *XXX* and the biological material from a slide biopsy, coded SB2;
- the reference sample from *XXX* and the post-surgery material included in a paraffin block, coded PB1.

Technical procedure

On the Nth day of Month, Year, Mr./Ms. *XXX* was present at *PPP* where he/she was identified by the presentation of a legally valid ID document, and filled and signed identification form *x* (copy attached, with a photograph taken at the collection site). Reference blood/saliva samples were taken under informed consent. Mr./Ms. *XXX* delivered also slide biopsies coded as SB1 and SB2, as well as a paraffin block coded as PB1.

Extracted genomic material (DNA) was amplified by PCR and analyzed after capillary electrophoresis using fragment size determination by automatic platforms (ABI PRISM 3130). The genetic markers analyzed are included in the kits Powerplex 16 HS (Promega Corporation) and Investigator ESSplex Plus (Qiagen).

The validated procedures used for storage, subsequent treatments, and analyses are described in the Internal Forms *ifx*, *ify*, *ifz* and *ifw* that are provided as appendices to this report. The results correspond to at least two independently performed analyses, by two different experts.

Results

Genotyping results are presented in Table 1. It was not possible to obtain complete genetic profiles for some duplicates of samples SB1 and SB2. This is likely due to DNA degradation, typical of this kind of material, which has been subject to extensive chemical treatments for their histological study.

Conclusions

The results obtained for 16 out of the 17 genetic markers analyzed, allows the conclusion that the genetic profile obtained from SB1 is distinct from the one observed in the reference sample. Therefore, it is possible to conclude that SB1 contains genetic material that can not have *XXX* as a contributor.

The genetic profiles obtained for the total number of genetic markers analyzed in SB2 (19) and PB1 (22) are identical to the one found in the reference sample from *XXX*. Therefore, it is not possible to exclude the hypothesis that *XXX* is the donor of the biological material present in SB2 and PB1.

Date and signatures

Table 1

Genetic markers	XXX (Reference sample)	SB1	SB2	PB1
CSF1PO	11–12	Nd	11–12	11–12
D1S1656	14–15	11	14–15	14–15
D2S1338	17–19	nd	nd	17–19
D2S441	10–11	13–14	10–11	10–11
D3S1358	18	14–16	18	18
D5S818	12–13	11	12–13	12–13
D7S820	9–10	8–12	9–10	9–10
D8S1179	11–15	13–14	11–15	11–15
D10S1248	14	13–15	14	14
D12S391	17	17–24	17	17
D13S317	11	11–12	11	11
D16S539	9–12	9–11	9–12	9–12
D18S51	15	16	15	15
D19S433	13–14	13.2–16.2	13–14	13–14
D21S11	27–28	30–34.2	27–28	27–28
D22S1045	15–16	11–15	15–16	15–16
FGA	22–25	nd	22–25	22–25
Penta D	11–12	nd	nd	11–12
Penta E	12–13	nd	nd	12–13
TH01	8	6–9.3	8	8
TPOX	8	8	8	8
vWA	16	15–17	16	16

nd: not determined.

II. Mock reports for paternity cases

This case corresponds to the Q&A 02:

"First-degree kinship (paternity/maternity): Is John Doe the Father of Ken?"

These reports correspond to situations in which the paternity/ maternity of an individual relative to another one is questioned, and both individuals—alleged father/mother and child—are available for testing. Using the standard, biparentally transmitted markers, paternity and maternity testing are equivalent and therefore, for simplicity's sake, and because it is the most commonly doubtful first-degree kinship, only paternity will be addressed afterwards.

In standard paternity cases, the alternative hypothesis to paternity is that the individuals alleged father and child are unrelated (i.e., the alleged father is unrelated to the mother of the child and there is no suspicion that the true father is related to the questioned one). The undoubted mother of the child may be unavailable for testing— case II.a., or otherwise—case II.b.

Complex paternity cases may involve situations where the alleged father may be related to the real one and thus, although not the father of the child, he is nonetheless paternally related to him/her—case II.c., or incestuous cases, where the alleged father is related to the mother of the child, and thus maternally related to him/her—case II.d.

II.a. *Standard putative father/child duo: Paternity not excluded*

Here we present the report on a standard paternity case in which the alleged father and the child are the only individuals available for analysis, sharing genetic information in all the markers typed, so that no incompatibility with transmission rules is observed. As previously mentioned, by a "standard paternity case" we mean that the individuals are either related as father-child or as unrelated.

Report II.a.

Paternity Test n° xx/yyyy

XXX asked for the genetic testing on the possible paternity relationship of

So-and-so

relatively to

Child

through the request ref. xxx (copy attached).

Technical procedure

On the Nth day of Month, Year, the individuals *So-and-so*, and *Child* were present at *PPP* where they were identified by the presentation of ID documents and filled and signed identification forms *x* and *y* (copies attached, containing photographs taken at the collection site).

Blood/saliva samples were taken. Storage and subsequent treatments and analyses were performed in the same way and under the same conditions. The validated procedures used for storage, subsequent treatments, and analyses are described in the Internal Forms *ifx*, *ify*, *ifz* and *ifw* that are provided as appendices to this report. Genetic profiles were made according to the specifications described in Annex 1 and correspond to at least two independent analyses, obtained also independently by two different experts.

Results

See Table 1.

Conclusions

Assuming the conditions described in Annex 2, the results obtained show that the genetic profiles configuration observed is **241,756,832** times (rounded up to a whole number) more likely assuming the hypothesis that So-and-so is the **biological father of Child** than under the hypothesis of the individuals being **genetically unrelated** (results per marker presented in Table 1).

Date and signatures

Table 1

Genetic markers	So-and-so	Child	Likelihood Ratios*
CSF1PO	12–13	10–12	0.804
D2S1338	24–25	19–24	2.488
D3S1358	14–16	14–15	2.420
D5S818	8–13	8–11	36.761
D7S820	10–12	10	1.889
D8S1179	11–12	11–14	2.663
D13S317	11–13	12–13	2.434
D16S539	11–13	13–14	1.376
D18S51	12–18	13–18	3.776
D19S433	13.2–15.2	13–13.2	32.048
D21S11	28–29	28–33.2	1.702
FGA	19–23	23	3.398
Penta D	2.2–8	8–11	12.137
Penta E	5–12	8–12	1.280
TH01	7–9	9	2.493
TPOX	8–11	8–11	1.369
VWA	16	16-18	2.171

* Rounded up to three decimals.

Date and signatures

Annex 1

Report II.a.

Paternity Test n° xx/yyyy

Genetic Markers and Methods

Genetic markers (or loci; singular: locus)

Genetic markers	Typing kit
CSF1PO	a,b
D1S1656	b
D2S1338	b
D2S441	b
D3S1358	a,b
D5S818	a
D7S820	a
D8S1179	a,b
D10S1248	b
D12S391	b
D13S317	a
D16S539	a,b
D18S51	a,b
D19S433	b
D21S11	a,b
D22S1045	b
FGA	a,b
Penta D	a
Penta E	a
TPOX	a
TH01	a,b
VWA	a,b

Methods

Genomic material (DNA) was extracted, amplified through PCR, and analyzed after capillary electrophoresis in an automatic sequencer (*equipment model and manufacturer*) according to the instructions from the manufacturers of kits a and b (*names and manufacturers*). All procedures are described in the Internal Forms *ixxx*. Considering the database X (*reference or description of the population sample used*) for allele frequencies, the *a priori* probability of two unrelated individuals sharing at least one allele for all the analyzed markers is equal to 1.065×10^{-06}. If the individuals are assumed as second-degree relatives (grandparent-grandchild, half-siblings, or avuncular), such probability equals 0.00338 (rounded up to five decimals).

Annex 2

Report II.a.

Paternity Test n° xx/yyyy

Theoretical, Statistical, and Probabilistic Framework

The approach used to weigh the evidentiary value of the results compares:

A – the probability of the observations (genetic profiles of the two individuals) assuming paternity,

and

B – the probability of the same observations assuming the two individuals are unrelated.

These hypotheses were, *a priori*, considered as equally likely by the requesting parties.

The comparison A/B takes the form of a Likelihood Ratio (LR, sometimes also designated as paternity index, PI), which measures how much the observed results are more likely under the hypothesis of paternity when compared to the alternative hypothesis, of no biological relationship.

The calculations are performed assuming that:

1. The putative father has no monozygotic ('identical') twin(s);
2. The putative father and the real father are genetically unrelated with the mother of the child;
3. The putative father is either the true father or genetically unrelated with him;
4. The tested individuals are assumed to belong to the population sampled for the estimation of gene frequencies (*reference and/or description of the population sample used, including sampling criteria*);
5. No gametic association (linkage disequilibrium) exists between the analyzed loci.

Calculations were performed using a home-developed software and confirmed using Software XXX, v. XXX, date, available at XXXX, using the parameters described below:

Allele Frequencies	[reference to the database employed]
Mutation model	Extended Stepwise Rate 1 = 0.001, Range = 0.1, Rate 2 = 10E-06 Females equal to males.
Allele lumping	Not considered.
Drop-in; Drop-out	Null
Coancestry coefficient	Null

All procedures are described in the Internal Forms *ifx*, *ify* and *ifz*, presented as appendices to this report.

II.b. Standard putative father/mother-child trio: Paternity practically excluded

In this case, we present a situation where, besides the alleged father and the child, the undoubted mother is also available for analysis. As before, the alleged father is unrelated with the mother of the child and the alleged father is either the true father or unrelated to him. A case is presented in which the genetic profile of the alleged father is extremely improbable under the hypothesis of paternity, being practically not compatible with those of the pair of the undoubted mother/child.

Report II.b.

Paternity Test n° xx/yyyy

XXX asked for the genetic testing on the possible paternity relationship of

So-and-so

relatively to

Child, undoubted son/daughter of Mother

through the request ref. xxx (copy attached).

Technical procedure

On the Nth day of Month, Year, the individuals *So-and-so*, *Mother* and *Child* were present at *PPP* where they were identified by the presentation of ID documents and filled and signed identification forms *x* and *y* (copies attached, containing photographs taken at the collection site).

Blood/saliva samples were taken. Storage and subsequent treatments and analyses were performed in the same way and under the same conditions. The validated procedures used for storage, subsequent treatments, and analyses are described in the Internal Forms *ifx*, *ify*, *ifz* and *ifw* that are provided as appendices to this report. Genetic profiles were made according to the specifications described in Annex 1 and correspond to at least two independent analyses, obtained also independently by two different experts.

Results

See Table 1.

Conclusions

Assuming the conditions described in Annex 2, the results obtained show that the observed genetic profiles are 2.06052×10^{-16} times more likely assuming the hypothesis that **So-and-so is the biological father of Child, undoubted son/daughter of Mother** than under the hypothesis of the **individuals So-and-So and Child being genetically unrelated** (results per marker presented in Table 1).

Conversely, the results obtained show that the observed genetic profiles are 4.85314×10^{15} times more likely assuming the hypothesis that **individuals So-and-So and Child, undoubted son/daughter of Mother, are genetically unrelated**, than under the hypothesis of the individuals being **related as father and child.**

Date and signatures

Table 1

Genetic markers	So-and-so	Child	Mother	Likelihood ratios[+]
CSF1PO	12–13	10–12	10–10	1.804
D2S1338*	24–25	23–24	24–27	0.099
D3S1358*	14–16	12–15	12–12	0.072
D5S818*	9–13	10–11	10–11	0.076
D7S820	10–12	10	10	1.889
D8S1179*	10–12	11–14	11–11	0.066
D13S317*	11–13	12–14	11–12	0.083
D16S539*	12–13	13–14	13–15	0.038
D18S51	12–18	13–18	13–13	3.786
D19S433*	13–15.2	14–15.2	15.2–15.2	0.048
D21S11*	29–29	28–33.2	28–29	0.070
FGA*	19–24	22	22–22	0.040
Penta D*	8–8	11–11	11–12	0.014
Penta E*	5–10	8–12	8–13	0.048
TH01	7–9	9	9–9	2.493
TPOX*	8–12	8–11	8–15	0.037
VWA*	17–19	16–18	16–20	0.017

[+] Rounded up to three decimals.
* Incompatibility with Mendelian transmission rules.

Date and signatures

Annex 1

Report II.b.

Paternity Test n° xx/yyyy

Genetic Markers and Methods

Genetic markers (or loci; singular: locus)

Genetic markers	Typing kit
CSF1PO	a,b
D1S1656	b
D2S1338	b
D2S441	b
D3S1358	a,b
D5S818	a
D7S820	a
D8S1179	a,b
D10S1248	b
D12S391	b
D13S317	a
D16S539	a,b
D18S51	a,b
D19S433	b
D21S11	a,b
D22S1045	b
FGA	a,b
Penta D	a
Penta E	a
TPOX	a
TH01	a,b
VWA	a,b

Methods

Genomic material (DNA) was extracted, amplified through PCR, and analyzed after capillary electrophoresis in an automatic sequencer (*equipment model and manufacturer*) according to the instructions from the manufacturers of kits a and b (*names and manufacturers*). All procedures are described in the Internal Forms *ixxx*. Considering the database X (*reference or description of the population sample used*) for allele frequencies the *a priori* probability of two unrelated individuals sharing at least one allele for all the analyzed markers is equal to 1.065×10^{-06}. If the individuals are assumed as second-degree relatives (grandparent-grandchild, half-siblings, or avuncular) such probability equals 0.00338 (rounded up to five decimals).

Annex 2

Report II.b.

Paternity Test n° xx/yyyy

Theoretical, Statistical, and Probabilistic Framework

The approach used to weight the evidentiary value of the results compares:

A – the probability of the observations (genetic profiles of the two individuals) assuming paternity,

and

B – the probability of the same observations assuming the two individuals are unrelated.

These hypotheses were, *a priori*, considered as equally likely by the requesting parties.

The comparison A/B takes the form of a Likelihood Ratio (LR, sometimes also designated as paternity index, PI), which therefore measures how much the observed results are more likely under the hypothesis of paternity when compared to the alternative hypothesis, of no biological relationship.

The calculations are performed assuming that:

1. The putative father has no monozygotic ('identical') twin(s);
2. The putative father and the real father are genetically unrelated with the mother of the child;
3. The putative father is either the true father or genetically unrelated with him;
4. The tested individuals are assumed to belong to the population sampled for the estimation of gene frequencies (*reference and/or description of the population sample used, including sampling criteria*);
5. No gametic association (linkage disequilibrium) exists between the analyzed loci.

Calculations were performed using a home developed software and confirmed using Software XXX, v. XXX, date, available at XXXX, using the parameters described below:

Allele Frequencies	[reference to the database employed]
Mutation model	Extended Stepwise Rate 1 = 0.001, Range = 0.1, Rate 2 = 10E-06 Females equal to males.
Allele lumping	Not considered.
Drop-in; Drop-out	Null
Coancestry coefficient	Null

All procedures are described in the Internal Forms *ifx*, *ify* and *ifz*, presented as appendices to this report.

II.c. Complex putative father/child duo: Putative father possibly related to the real one

Here we describe and analyze the situation where, after a standard paternity case report was issued to the court (in which the genetic profiles were much more likely under the hypothesis of paternity than under the unrelated one), it was returned with the new information that the man, refusing paternity, claims that the true father is in fact his deceased full brother. Mock report II.c. concerns a duo case where a first paternity report was issued and then returned with the added information that the putative father claims that the true father is his (unavailable) brother.

We will discuss how to deal with this added information, which creates a situation where, under the assumption of one of the hypotheses of kinship, the alleged father—the deceased full brother—is not available for testing.

Now, the possibility of the real father of the child to be the unavailable full brother of the tested individual needs to be evaluated. Therefore, what will be possible to analyze, instead of paternity, is an avuncular relationship, that is, what is the likelihood of so-and-so to be an uncle of the child.

When general kinship analyses are made, it must be clarified and clearly transmitted in the report that when using the routine kits of unassociated biparentally transmitted genetic markers, what is possible is to distinguish between classes of pedigrees, not between pedigrees themselves. Indeed, distinct pedigrees, if belonging to the same class, provide the same numerical value for the quantification of the evidence (Thompson 1976, Weir et al. 2006, Pinto et al. 2010). In favorable cases, however, some of these pedigrees can be ruled out, considering other sources of information than genetics, such as age, death before the period of conception of the child, and so on.

Indeed, in the framework of paternity analyses, where two or even three individuals (putative father, child and, possibly, the mother of the child) are typed, it is equally likely the real father of the child to be (a.) a full-brother, (b.) the father, or (c.) a son, of the tested alleged father, since the three pedigrees: (a.) avuncular, (b.) half-siblings, and (c.) grandparent-grandchild, belong to (and compose) a specific autosomal kinship class of pedigrees and are, therefore, indistinguishable through autosomal unassociated markers. Below the scheme depicting the second-degree pedigrees belonging to the same kinship class:

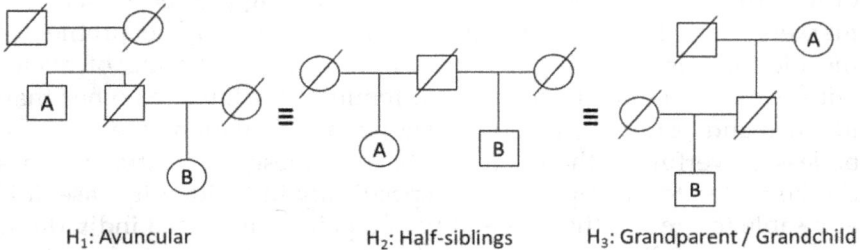

H_1: Avuncular H_2: Half-siblings H_3: Grandparent / Grandchild

Note that, regardless of the amount of unassociated autosomal data analyzed, the pedigrees are (theoretically) indistinguishable. Indeed,

$$LR = \frac{P(G \mid H_1)}{P(G \mid H_2)} = \frac{P(G \mid H_1)}{P(G \mid H_3)} = \frac{P(G \mid H_2)}{P(G \mid H_3)} = 1, \text{ for any genetic configuration}$$

G and assuming the a priori probabilities $P(H_i)$, for i = 1, 2, 3, as equally likely.

Thus, to quantify the possibility of the tested individuals being related as uncle- nephew/niece, the possibility of the real father of the child to be the father or a son of the tested man (in which cases the individuals are related as half-siblings and grandfather-grandchild, respectively) must be discarded *a priori* (based upon sources of information other than genetics).

Technical, statistical, and probabilistic framework

Note that techniques, methods, assumptions, and even the genetic materials sampled are the same for this second analysis, assuming the individuals related as uncle-nephew/niece and no extra genetic analyses in the wet laboratory are required. Indeed, only the theoretical framework of the case has changed, and solely new statistical calculations are needed. As discussed previously, only autosomal, unlinked, and unassociated markers, expected to be in conformity with Hardy-Weinberg expectations, are considered. Reliable estimates for allele frequencies and mutation rates are (again) assumed to be available.

Particularly for the cases where other possibilities beyond identity and paternity are involved, experts should consider the possibility of including in the report parameters concerning the set of analyzed markers (and thus ensure they are independent of the profiles of the individuals of a specific case). Indeed, since sharing of alleles with the same familial origin is not required for kinships other than identity and paternity/maternity, statistical calculations are likely to be less powerful for the pedigrees beyond these, and extra statistics can be added to the report. Then, specifically in an identity case, it is advisable to present the probability of a pair of unrelated individuals and a pair of full siblings having the same genetic profile for all the analyzed markers. Changes in these hypotheses may be performed depending on the case in question—for example, both father and child being suspects of the same crime.

When dealing with a questioned paternity the probability of a pair of unrelated individuals and a pair of second-degree relatives sharing at least one allele for all the markers is recommended (algebraic formulae are found in Weir et al. 2006, and Pinto et al. 2013). These statistics should be presented in the report as well as the description of genetic markers and methods used, evidencing their independence from the specific case analyzed.

Formulation of propositions

Hypotheses of kinship here considered are as follows and assumed to be exhaustive and mutually exclusive, according to the court's new scenario.

H1: The profiles correspond to a pair of individuals related as father/child.

H2: The profiles correspond to a pair of individuals related as avuncular.

The quantitative evaluation is presented on the report as follows:

1. The probability of the observations (genetic profiles) under H1;
2. The probability of the observations (genetic profiles) under H2;
3. A Likelihood Ratio between probabilities 1. and 2.

References

Pinto, N., Silva, P.V. and Amorim, A. (2010). General derivation of the sets of pedigrees with the same kinship coefficients. Hum Hered., 70: 194–204.

Pinto, N., Gusmão, L., Egeland, T. and Amorim, A. (2013). Paternity exclusion power: Comparative behaviour of autosomal and X-chromosomal markers in standard and deficient cases with inbreeding. Forensic Sci. Int. Genet., 7(2): 290–5.

Thompson, E. (1975). The estimation of pairwise relationships. Ann. Hum Genet., 39: 173–188.

Weir, B.S., Anderson, A.D. and Hepler, A.B. (2006). Genetic relatedness analysis: Modern data and new challenges. Nat. Rev. Genet., 7: 771–780.

Report II.c.

Kinship Test n° xx/yyyy

The *XXXX* asked for the genetic testing on the possible avuncular relationship of

So-and-so

relatively to

Child

through the request ref. *xxx* (copy attached), assuming that the alternative kinship is paternity.

Technical procedures

On the Nth of Month, Year, both individuals were present at the Institute/Laboratory *PPP* where they were identified by presentation of ID documents and filled and signed the identification forms *x* and *y* (copy attached, containing photographs taken at the collection site). Blood/saliva samples were taken. Storage, and subsequent treatments and analyses were performed in the same way and under the same conditions. Genetic profiles were made according to the specifications described in Annex 1 and correspond to at least two results obtained independently by two experts.

On the Nth of Month, Year, a report was issued statistically comparing the probabilities of the genetic configuration of the individuals assuming the hypotheses: A - The two profiles correspond to a pair of individuals related as parent/child, and B - The two profiles correspond to a pair of genetically unrelated individuals. A result favoring paternity was obtained – see Report (II.a.) attached.

On the Nth of Month, Year, the up mentioned report was returned with the information that So-and-So refuses the paternity, claiming that the true father is in fact his meanwhile deceased full brother. New statistical calculations accommodating this information and the hypotheses: A – the two profiles correspond to a pair of individuals related as parent/child, and C – the two profiles correspond to a pair of individuals related as avuncular, were computed.

Results

See Table 1.

Conclusions

Assuming the conditions described in Annex 2, the results obtained show that the genetic profile configuration is 306 times (rounded up to units) more probable assuming the hypothesis that So-and-so is the biological father of Child than under the hypothesis of the individuals being related as uncle-nephew (numerical results per marker presented in Table 1).

Date and signatures

Report II.c.

Paternity vs. Avuncularity Test

n° xx/yyyy

Table 1

Genetic markers	So-and-so	Child	Likelihood ratios*
CSF1PO	12–13	10–12	0.891
D2S1338	24–25	19–24	1.427
D3S1358	14–16	14–15	1.415
D5S818	8–13	8–11	1.947
D7S820	10–12	10	1.308
D8S1179	11–12	11–14	1.454
D13S317	11–13	12–13	1.418
D16S539	11–13	13–14	1.158
D18S51	12–18	13–18	1.581
D19S433	13.2–15.2	13–13.2	1.939
D21S11	28–29	28–33.2	1.260
FGA	19–23	23	1.545
Penta D	2.2–8	8–11	1.848
Penta E	5–12	8–12	1.123
TH01	7–9	9	1.427
TPOX	8–11	8–11	1.156
VWA	16	16–18	1.369

* Rounded up to three decimals.

Annex 1

Report II.c.

Test nº xx/yyyy

Genetic Markers and Methods

Genetic markers (or loci; singular: locus)

Genetic markers	Typing kit
CSF1PO	a,b
D1S1656	b
D2S1338	b
D2S441	b
D3S1358	a,b
D5S818	a
D7S820	a
D8S1179	a,b
D10S1248	b
D12S391	b
D13S317	a
D16S539	a,b
D18S51	a,b
D19S433	b
D21S11	a,b
D22S1045	b
FGA	a,b
Penta D	a
Penta E	a
TPOX	a
TH01	a,b
VWA	a,b

Methods

Genomic material (DNA) was extracted, amplified through PCR, and analyzed after capillary electrophoresis in an automatic sequencer (*equipment model and manufacturer*) according to the instructions from the manufacturers' kits a and b (*names and manufacturers*). All procedures are described in the Internal Forms *xxx*. Considering the database X (*reference or description of the population sample used*) for allele frequencies, the *a priori* probability of two unrelated individuals sharing at least one allele for all the analyzed markers is equal to $1.065E \times 10^{-06}$. If the individuals are assumed as second-degree relatives (grandparent-grandchild, half-siblings or avuncular) such probability equals 0.00338 (rounded up to five decimals).

Annex 2

Report II.c.

Test n° xx/yyyy

Theoretical, Statistical, and Probabilistic Framework

The approach used to weight the evidentiary value of the results compares:

A – The probability of the observations (genetic profiles of the two individuals) assuming paternity,

and

C – The probability of the same observations assuming the putative father as full-brother of the real one.

These hypotheses were, *a priori*, considered as equally likely by the requesting parties.

The comparisons A/C take the form of likelihood ratios (LRs) which therefore measure how much the observed genetic results are more probable under the hypothesis of paternity relative to the alternative hypothesis of avuncularity.

The calculations are performed assuming that:

1. The putative father has no monozygotic ('identical') twin(s).
2. The probabilities of the hypotheses of the putative father to be the father or son of the real father are *a priori* considered as nil.
3. The putative father and the real father are genetically unrelated with the mother of the child.
4. The putative father is either: (a.) the true father, or (b.) a full brother of him.
5. The tested individuals are assumed to belong to the population sampled for the estimation of gene frequencies (*reference and/*

or description of the population sample used, including the sampling criteria).

6. No gametic association (linkage disequilibrium) exists between the analyzed loci.

Calculations were performed using Software XXX, v. XXX, date, available at XXXX.

Allele Frequencies	[reference to the database employed]
Mutation model	Extended Stepwise Rate 1 = 0.001, Range = 0.1, Rate 2 = 10E-06 Females equal to males.
Allele lumping	Not considered.
Drop-in; Drop-out	Null
Coancestry coefficient	Null

All procedures are described in the Internal Forms XXX and YYY.

II.d. Complex putative father/mother-child trio: The putative father is related to the mother of the child

Here we describe and analyze the situation of a paternity testing where the alleged father of the child is related to his/her undoubted mother. This type of forensics analysis may arise in criminal situations of sexual abuse, for example, but also in civil litigations — the alleged father and undoubted mother related as full first cousins (the father/mother of one is full-sibling of the father/mother of the other), for example. In any case, the existing relationship must be properly reported and included in the computations, even if the mother of the child is not available for analysis.

If the alleged father is tested, the corresponding reports are essentially similar to Reports II.a. (undoubted mother unavailable) and II.b. (or otherwise), once the formulation of the propositions are well established and the hypotheses of relationship between the individuals (main H1, or alternative H2) clearly defined. For example:

H1: The alleged father, undoubted father of the undoubted mother, is the father of the child.

H2: The alleged father, undoubted father of the undoubted mother, is unrelated with the father of the child.

Or,

H1: The alleged father, undoubted full first cousin of the undoubted mother, is the father of the child.

H2: The alleged father, undoubted full first cousin of the undoubted mother, is unrelated with the father of the child.

In any case it should be clear that the number of homozygosities (situation of two identical alleles at a marker) observed in the offspring of two related individuals is expectedly higher than the one observed on the offspring of two unrelated ones (increasingly higher as closer is the relationship between the mother and the father of the child). As before, the quantitative evaluation of the evidence is presented on the report via the computation of a likelihood ratio between the probabilities of the observations (genetic profiles) assuming the alternative hypotheses, if priors are not considered. In the herein presented mock report, a trio paternity case where the alleged father is half-brother of the mother is considered.

Report II.d.

Paternity Test n° xx/yyyy

XXX asked for the genetic testing on the possible paternity relationship of

So-and-so

relatively to

Child, undoubted son/daughter of Mother, undoubted half-sister of So-and-So,

through the request ref. xxx (copy attached).

Technical procedure

On the Nth day of Month, Year, the individuals *So-and-so, Mother,* and *Child* were present at *PPP* where they were identified by the presentation of ID documents and filled and signed identification forms *x* and *y* (copies attached, containing photographs taken at the collection site).

Blood/saliva samples were taken; storage and subsequent treatments and analyses were performed in the same way and under the same conditions. The validated procedures used for storage, subsequent treatments, and analyses are described in the Internal Forms *ifx, ify, ifz,* and *ifw* that are provided as appendices to this report. Genetic profiles were made according to the specifications described in Annex 1 and correspond to at least two independent analyses, obtained independently by two different experts.

Results

See Table 1.

Conclusions

Assuming the conditions described in Annex 2, specifically that *So-and-So* is half-brother of the *Mother*, the results obtained show that the genetic profiles configuration observed is 80,816,687 times (rounded up to a whole number), more likely assuming the hypothesis that So-and-so is the **biological father of the Child, rather** than the hypothesis of the **father being an individual genetically unrelated to him** (results per marker presented in Table 1).

Date and signatures

Table 1

Genetic markers	So-and-so	Child	Mother	Likelihood ratios[+]
CSF1PO	12–13	10–12	10–12	2.803
D2S1338	24–25	24–25	24–27	3.099
D3S1358	14–16	14	14–12	3.076
D5S818	10–13	10–11	10–11	5.033
D7S820	10–12	10	10	2.889
D8S1179	14–12	11–14	11–11	1.166
D13S317	13–14	12–14	11–12	2.094
D16S539	12–13	13	13–15	2.085
D18S51	12–18	13–18	13–13	3.786
D19S433	14–15.2	14–15.2	15.2–15.2	6.046
D21S11	29–29	28–29	28–29	3.708
FGA	19–22	22	22–22	2.030
Penta D	8–8	8–11	11–12	5.014
Penta E	5–10	8–10	8–13	3.246
TH01	9–9	9	9–9	1.453
TPOX	8–12	8	8–15	2.746
VWA	16–19	16	16–20	3.652

[+] Rounded up to three decimals.

Date and signatures

Annex 1

Report II.d.

Test n° xx/yyyy

Genetic Markers and Methods

Genetic markers (or loci; singular: locus)

Genetic markers	Typing kit
CSF1PO	a,b
D1S1656	b
D2S1338	b
D2S441	b
D3S1358	a,b
D5S818	a
D7S820	a
D8S1179	a,b
D10S1248	b
D12S391	b
D13S317	a
D16S539	a,b
D18S51	a,b
D19S433	b
D21S11	a,b
D22S1045	b
FGA	a,b
Penta D	a
Penta E	a
TPOX	a
TH01	a,b
VWA	a,b

Methods

Genomic material (DNA) was extracted, amplified through PCR, and analyzed after capillary electrophoresis in an automatic sequencer (*equipment model and manufacturer*), according to the instructions from the manufacturers' kits a and b (*names and manufacturers*). All procedures are described in the Internal Forms *xxx*. Considering the database X (*reference or description of the population sample used*) for allele frequencies, the *a priori* probability of two unrelated individuals share at least one allele for all the analyzed markers is equal to 1.065×10^{-06}. If the individuals are assumed as second-degree relatives (grandparent-grandchild, half-siblings or avuncular) such probability equals 0.00338 (rounded up to five decimals).

Annex 2

Report II.d.

Test n° xx/yyyy

Theoretical, Statistical, and Probabilistic Framework

The approach used to weight the evidentiary value of the results compares:

A – the probability of the observations (genetic profiles of the two individuals) assuming paternity,

and

B – the probability of the same observations assuming that the real father and the analyzed alleged father are unrelated.

These hypotheses were, *a priori*, considered as equally likely by the requesting parties.

The comparison A/B takes the form of a Likelihood Ratio (LR, sometimes also designated as paternity index, PI) which therefore measures how much the observed results are more likely under the hypothesis of paternity when compared to the alternative hypothesis, of no biological relationship between the real and the analyzed alleged father.

The calculations are performed assuming that:

1. The putative father has no monozygotic ('identical') twin(s);
2. The putative father is half-brother of the mother;
3. The real father is either the putative father or an individual genetically unrelated with both the putative father and the mother of the child;
4. The tested individuals are assumed to belong to the population sampled for the estimation of gene frequencies (*reference and/or description of the population sample used, including sampling criteria*);
5. No gametic association (linkage disequilibrium) exists between the analyzed loci.

Calculations were performed using Software XXX, v. XXX, date, available at XXXX, using the parameters described below:

Allele Frequencies	[reference to the database employed]
Mutation model	Extended Stepwise Rate 1 = 0.001, Range = 0.1, Rate 2 = 10E-06 Females equal to males.
Allele lumping	Not considered.
Drop-in; Drop-out	Null
Coancestry coefficient	Null

All procedures are described in the Internal Forms *ifx*, *ify*, and *ifz*, presented as appendices to this report.

III. Mock reports for complex kinship cases

This case corresponds to the Q&A 03:

"Other kinships: are John and Bill related as, for instance, sibs?"

These reports correspond to situations where other kinships, beyond identity and paternity/maternity, need to be evaluated. Once the father/mother in question is not available for analysis, these are, by nature, much more complex problems. Also, as the sharing of alleles with a common familial ancestral is not mandatory in this type of relationship, the statistical significance of the results is weaker than in those obtained for identity and paternity/maternity. Indeed, results are much more dependent on the parameters used, as is the case of the allele frequency population database, depending the statistical significance of the results on the problem in question, the individuals analyzed, and their genotypes. The problems here addressed concern a full-sibship problem (case III.a.), and a putative case of incest where the alleged father is not available for testing (case III.b.).

III.a. Sibship problem

Regarding sibship problems, the standard analyses rely on the comparison of the probability of the observations under the following hypotheses: *(i)* full-siblings *versus* half-siblings—when there is no doubt that the individuals share the same mother, contrary to what occurs for the father, *(ii)* full-siblings versus unrelated—e.g., in the case of victims' identification in mass disasters, or *(iii)* half-siblings *versus* unrelated – when individuals, knowing to have different mothers, want to evaluate the possibility of sharing the same father.

The herein presented mock report concerns the situation *(i)*, where a male/female pair requires the evaluation of the possibility of being offspring of the same father, knowing they have the same mother. It is noteworthy that if they were two males, the analysis of Y chromosomal markers could provide important insights in this case, as paternal brothers share such genotypic information unless mutation occurs. In this case, as a female is involved, biparentally transmitted markers are required to be analyzed.

Since the sharing of alleles with the same familial ancestry is not required for the kinship hypotheses under consideration, the computation of simulations to understand the expected distribution of the results in the population may be of help. If experts opt to provide this information, it should be clearly reported that it concerns the population itself (allele frequencies), regardless of the genotypic configuration of the analyzed individuals, i.e., is population, not case, specific.

Report III.a.

Full-Sibship Test n° xx/yyyy

XXX asked for the genetic testing on the possible full-sibship relationship of

> Ms. So-and-so

relatively to

> Mister So-and-so, her undoubted maternal brother,

through the request ref. xxx (copy attached).

Technical procedure

On the Nth day of Month, Year, the individuals *Ms. So-and-so*, and *Mister So-and-so* were present at *PPP* where they were identified by the presentation of ID documents and filled and signed identification forms *x* and *y* (copies attached, containing photographs taken at the collection site).

Blood/saliva samples were taken. Storage and subsequent treatments and analyses were performed in the same way and under the same conditions. The validated procedures used for storage, subsequent treatments, and analyses are described in the Internal Forms *ifx*, *ify*, *ifz*, and *ifw* that are provided as appendices to this report. Genetic profiles were made according to the specifications described in Annex 1 and correspond to at least two independent analyses, obtained also independently by two different experts.

Results

See Table 1.

Conclusions

Assuming the conditions described in Annex 2, and that *Mister So-and-So* is half-brother of *Miss So-and-so*, the results obtained show that the genetic profiles configuration observed is 6,082 times (rounded up to a whole number), more likely assuming the hypothesis that *Mister So-and-So* is full brother of the *Miss So-and-so*, than the hypothesis of them being half sibs (results per marker presented in Table 1).

Date and signatures

Table 1

Genetic markers	*Ms. So-and-so*	*Mister So-and-So*	Likelihood ratios+
D3S1358	14, 16	14, 16	2.028
VWA	17,11	17,11	2.469
D16S539	11, 13	11	0.805
CSF1PO	11, 12	11, 12	0.731
TPOX	8, 11	8	1.542
D8S1179	12, 13	11, 13	2.822
D21S11	28, 32.2	28, 32.2	3.845
D18S51	13, 14	13, 14	3.843
D2S441	10, 11	10, 11	2.207
D19S433	13, 14	13, 16	0.733
TH01	9	6, 9	0.851
FGA	20, 22	21	0.5
D22S1045	11, 16	11, 15	0.866
D5S818	11	11	1.988
D13S317	11, 12	11, 12	1.834
D7S820	6.3, 11	10	0.5
SE33	16, 21	16, 27.2	0.905
D10S1248	15, 17	16, 17	0.946
D1S1656	12	12	3.316
D12S391	20, 23	18.3, 22	0.5

D2S1338	17, 25	17, 19	0.743
Penta E	5, 12	12	0.861
Penta D	11, 14	10, 11	0.784
D7S1517	24, 25	25	0.858
D3S1744	18, 20	18, 20	5.193
D2S1360	22	22	2.622
D6S474	14, 16	16	0.812
D4S2366	10, 12	10	0.885
D8S1132	19, 23	19, 23	3.976
D5S2500	15	12, 15	0.840
D21S2055	34, 37	19.1, 26	0.5
D10S2325	11	11	3.136

⁺Rounded up to 3 decimals.

Date and signatures

Annex 1

Report III.a.

Test n° xx/yyyy

Genetic Markers and Methods

Genetic markers (or loci; singular: locus)

Genetic markers	Typing kit
D3S1358	a,b
VWA	a,b
D16S539	a,b
CSF1PO	a,b
TPOX	a,b
D8S1179	a,b
D21S11	a,b
D18S51	a,b
D2S441	a,b
D19S433	a,b
TH01	a,b
FGA	a,b
D22S1045	a,b
D5S818	a,b
D13S317	a,b
D7S820	a,b
SE33	a,b
D10S1248	a,b
D1S1656	a,b
D12S391	a,b
D2S1338	a,b
Penta E	b
Penta D	b

D7S1517	c
D3S1744	c
D2S1360	c
D6S474	c
D4S2366	c
D8S1132	c
D5S2500	c
D21S2055	c
D10S2325	c

Methods

Genomic material (DNA) was extracted, amplified through PCR, and analyzed after capillary electrophoresis in an automatic sequencer (*equipment model and manufacturer*) according to the instructions from the manufacturers' kits a, b, and c (*names and manufacturers*). All procedures are described in the Internal Forms *xxx*.

Annex 2

Report III.a.

Test n° xx/yyyy

Theoretical, Statistical, and Probabilistic Framework

The approach used to weight the evidentiary value of the results compares:

A – the probability of the observations (genetic profiles of the two individuals) assuming full-sibship,

and

B – the probability of the same observations assuming that the individuals are maternal half-siblings, the corresponding fathers being unrelated.

These hypotheses were, *a priori*, considered as equally likely by the requesting parties.

The comparison A/B takes the form of a Likelihood Ratio (LR) which therefore measures how much the observed results are more likely under the hypothesis of full-sibship when compared to the alternative hypothesis of maternal half-sibship between the analyzed individuals.

The calculations are performed assuming that:

1. The individuals share the same mother;
2. The father of the tested individuals is either the same individual or a pair of unrelated individuals;
3. The tested individuals are assumed to belong to the population sampled for the estimation of gene frequencies (*reference and/or description of the population sample used, including sampling criteria*);
4. No gametic association (linkage disequilibrium) exists between the analyzed loci.

179

Calculations were performed using Software XXX, v. XXX, date, available at XXXX, using the parameters described below:

Allele Frequencies	[reference to the databases employed]
Mutation model	Null
Allele lumping	Not considered.
Drop-in; Drop-out	Null
Coancestry coefficient	Null

Under the same assumptions and using the same software XXX, v. XXX, 10,000 pairs of genotypic configurations were randomly simulated (seed: 1234), assuming hypotheses A and B. The summary of the curves corresponding to the obtained likelihood ratio values is presented below:

Kinship Hypotheses	Likelihood Ratio				
	Median	Average	95%	5%	Standard Deviation
A true	1402	1.202E+07	2.073E+06	1.388	3.49E+08
B true	0.003496	0.7133	0.5861	5.009 E-05	21.19

From these, the proportion of cases for which a likelihood ratio greater than 6,082 was obtained reached 36.8600% when simulated hypothesis A, and 0.0000% when simulated hypothesis B (false positives).

All procedures are described in the Internal Forms *ifx*, *ify*, and *ifz*, presented as appendices to this report.

III.b. Incest problem: Alleged and absent father related to the mother of the child

The relation existing between the mother and the father of a child may be evaluated even without directly analyzing him or her. Indeed, the mock report here presented will focus on a putative case of incest where the alleged father, father of the mother, is not available for analysis. This scenario may arise for example in the investigative phase of a case of sexual abuse, which resulted in the conception of a child (or fetus) with a high number of homozygosities (situation of identical alleles at many markers). Typically, this investigation emerges in situations where a female with Down syndrome shows up pregnant, and the possibility of proceeding with an abortion is evaluated. The possibility of the father of the child being closely related with her can then emerge.

As before, the existence of pedigrees belonging to the same kinship class should be considered. Indeed, if the alleged father is not available for testing, the genotypic observations are equally likely if the father of the child is either the father, or a full brother (or even another son) of the mother. Such alternative kinship hypotheses should thus be excluded, considering other factors than genetics, before data evaluation. In the case that none of the hypotheses can be excluded, experts and laypersons must be aware that they are theoretically impossible to distinguish, regardless the amount of data regarding independent markers analyzed.

Report III.b.

Incest Test n° xx/yyyy

XXX asked for the genetic testing on the possible paternity of the father of

> Ms. So-and-So,

relatively to her fetus,

through the request ref. xxx (copy attached), where it is stated that Ms. So-and-So has Down syndrome.

Technical procedure

On the Nth day of Month, Year, blood reference samples from *Miss So-and-so*, and her fetus were received at *PPP* (chain of custody documentation annexed). *Miss So-and-so* was referred as affected by Down syndrome (clinical documentation annexed to the request).

Storage and subsequent treatments and analyses were performed in the same way and under the same conditions. The validated procedures used for storage, subsequent treatments, and analyses are described in the Internal Forms *ifx*, *ify*, *ifz*, and *ifw* that are provided as appendices to this report. Genetic profiles were made according to the specifications described in Annex 1 and correspond to at least two independent analyses, obtained also independently by two different experts. Markers D21S11, Penta D, and D21S2055 were excluded from the analyses due to the trisomy of *Ms. So-and-so*.

Results

See Table 1.

Conclusions

Assuming the conditions described in Annex 2, specifically that the alleged and absent father is the father of the mother of the fetus, the results obtained show that the genetic profiles configuration observed is 177,939 times (rounded up to a whole number), more likely assuming the hypothesis that the father of the fetus is the father of the mother, than under the hypothesis of mother and father being unrelated (results per marker presented in Table 1).

Date and signatures

Table 1

Genetic markers	*Ms. So-and-so*	*Fetus*	Likelihood ratios+
D3S1358	15, 16	15, 16	1.426
VWA	17, 17	17, 17	2.469
D16S539	11, 12	11, 11	1.281
CSF1PO	10, 12	12, 12	1.356
TPOX	8, 11	11, 11	1.426
D8S1179	11, 13	11, 13	1.763

D18S51	13, 14	13, 14	2.366
D2S441	10, 11	10, 11	1.519
D19S433	13, 14	13, 16	0.500
TH01	9, 9	6, 9	0.500
FGA	20, 22	20, 20	2.423
D22S1045	11, 16	11, 15	0.5
D5S818	11, 11	11, 11	1.988
D13S317	11, 12	12, 12	1.454
D7S820	7, 11	11, 11	1.626
SE33	16, 21	16, 27.2	0.5
D10S1248	15, 17	15, 17	3.266
D1S1656	12, 12	12, 12	3.316
D12S391	20, 23	20, 22	0.5
D2S1338	17, 25	17, 17	1.447
Penta E	5, 12	12, 12	1.802
D7S1517	24, 25	25, 25	1.697
D3S1744	18, 20	20, 20	7.080
D2S1360	22, 22	22, 22	2.199
D6S474	14, 16	16, 16	1.388
D4S2366	10, 12	10, 10	2.256
D8S1132	19, 23	19, 23	2.403
D5S2500	15, 15	12, 15	0.5
D10S2325	11, 11	11, 11	3.225

⁺Rounded up to three decimals.

Date and signatures

Annex 1

Report III.b.

Test n° xx/yyyy

Genetic Markers and Methods

Genetic markers (or loci; singular: locus)

Genetic markers	Typing kit
D3S1358	a,b
VWA	a,b
D16S539	a,b
CSF1PO	a,b
TPOX	a,b
D8S1179	a,b
D21S11*	a,b
D18S51	a,b
D2S441	a,b
D19S433	a,b
TH01	a,b
FGA	a,b
D22S1045	a,b
D5S818	a,b
D13S317	a,b
D7S820	a,b
SE33	a,b
D10S1248	a,b
D1S1656	a,b
D12S391	a,b
D2S1338	a,b
Penta E	b
Penta D*	b

D7S1517	c
D3S1744	c
D2S1360	c
D6S474	c
D4S2366	c
D8S1132	c
D5S2500	c
D21S2055*	c
D10S2325	c

Methods

Genomic material (DNA) was extracted, amplified through PCR, and analyzed after capillary electrophoresis in an automatic sequencer (*equipment model and manufacturer*), according to the instructions from the manufacturers' kits a, b, and c (*names and manufacturers*). All procedures are described in the Internal Forms *xxx*. *Markers located in the chromosome 21 are not considered in the analysis due to the trisomy of the analyzed individual.

Annex 2

Report III.b.

Test n° xx/yyyy

Theoretical, Statistical, and Probabilistic Framework

The approach used to weight the evidentiary value of the results compares:

A – the probability of the observations (genetic profiles of the two individuals) assuming that the father of the fetus is the father of the mother,

and

B – the probability of the same observations assuming that the father and the mother of the fetus are unrelated.

These hypotheses were, *a priori*, considered as equally likely by the requesting parties.

The comparison A/B takes the form of a Likelihood Ratio (LR) which therefore measures how much the observed results are more likely under the hypothesis of the father of the mother being also the father of the fetus when compared to the alternative hypothesis of father and mother being unrelated individuals.

The calculations are performed assuming that:

1. The putative father has no monozygotic ('identical') twin(s);
2. The putative father is either the true father or genetically unrelated with him;
3. A full-brother or any other son of the mother were *a priori* excluded to be the father of the fetus;
4. The tested individuals are assumed to belong to the population sampled for the estimation of gene frequencies (*reference and/or description of the population sample used, including sampling criteria*);
5. No gametic association (linkage disequilibrium) exists between the analyzed loci.

Calculations were performed using Software XXX, v. XXX, date, available at XXXX, using the parameters described below:

Allele Frequencies	[reference to the databases employed]
Mutation model	Null
Allele lumping	Not considered.
Drop-in; Drop-out	Null
Coancestry coefficient	Null

Under the same assumptions and using the same software XXX, v. XXX, 10,000 pairs of genotypic configurations were randomly simulated (seed: 1234), assuming hypotheses A and B. The summary of the curves corresponding to the obtained likelihood ratio values is presented below:

Kinship Hypotheses	Likelihood Ratio				
	Median	Average	95%	5%	Standard Deviation
A true	5,529	8.875E+07	8.106E+06	4.087	6.225E+09
B true	0.0004935	0.3748	0.2115	2.246 E-06	10.02

From these, the proportion of cases for which a likelihood ratio greater than 177,939 was obtained reached 21.6200% when hypothesis A was simulated, and 0.0000% when hypothesis B was simulated (false positives).

All procedures are described in the Internal Forms *ifx*, *ify*, and *ifz*, presented as appendices to this report.

IV. Mock report for a case of species identification

This case corresponds to the Q&A

1. Taxonomic identification: *Is this item from a given species?*

7.a. Does this item contain material from the protected species X?

Report

Species identification Test n° xx/yyyy

The XXX requested the identification of the fish species present in a shipment consisting frozen fish filets in boxes labelled as "haddock".

Technical procedures

Under XXX request, on the day/month/year, S, the expert from the Lab made the sample collection in the storage room where the questioned materials were.

In the same day, the barcoding identified (N°s 10213240 a 10213245) sealed bags containing the samples were custodied to the lab. Each bag corresponded to one pallet sampled, and from each pallet two boxes of frozen fish filets were randomly chosen (except in the case of 10213244, in which just one box was sampled as the corresponding pallet was half-empty). Inside each box, two pieces were collected, also aleatorily, and stored in separate tubes. In total, 22 samples were collected, from 11 boxes belonging to 6 pallets.

For genetic testing, one randomly chosen sample from each box was used. Processing and storage procedures and conditions were the same for all samples.

Genetic analyses were performed after specific PCR amplification of the DNA barcode region at the mitochondrial cytochrome c oxidase, subunit I (COI), using a primers' cocktail according to the references below (Ivanova et al. 2007, Ward et al. 2005); amplification products were submitted to Sanger sequencing. Resulting sequences were analyzed and edited using Geneious R7 (v. 7.0.6) software. Sequence Alignments and searches for similarities were performed with BLAST (*Basic Local Alignment Search Tool*) (http://blast.ncbi.nlm.nih.gov/ Blast.cgi?PROGRAM=blastn&PAGE_TYPE=BlastSearch&LINK_ LOC=blasthome) and BOLDSystems (*The Barcode of Life Data Systems*) (http://www.boldsystems.org/index.php/IDS_OpenIdEngine).

Results

Displayed in Table 1.

Conclusions

The obtained results allow the conclusion that in 10 out of the sampled boxes, DNA with a sequence identical to *Gadus morhua* ("codfish") was found, whereas in just one the DNA sequence corresponds to the label ("haddock", *Melanogrammus aeglefinus*).

Date and signatures

Table 1

Pallet N°	Box N°	DNA sequence interpretation [3] (% identity)
10213240	1	100% *Gadus morhua* (codfish)
	2	100% *Gadus morhua* (codfish)
10213241	1	100% *Gadus morhua* (codfish)
	2	100% *Gadus morhua* (codfish)
10213242	1	100% *Gadus morhua* (codfish)
	2	100% *Gadus morhua* (codfish)
10213243	1	100% *Gadus morhua* (codfish)
	2	100% *Gadus morhua* (codfish)
10213244	1	100% *Gadus morhua* (codfish)
10213245	1	100% *Melanogrammus aeglefinus* (haddock)
	2	100% *Gadus morhua* (codfish)
Total: 6	Total: 11	

References

Ivanova, N.V. et al. (2007). Universal primer cocktails for fish DNA barcoding. Molecular Ecology Notes, 7(4): 544–548.

http://blast.ncbi.nlm.nih.gov/Blast.cgi?PROGRAM=blastn&PAGE_TYPE=BlastSearch&LINK_LOC=blasthome.

http://www.boldsystems.org/index.php/IDS_OpenIdEngine.

Ward, R.D. et al. (2005). DNA barcoding Australia's fish species. Philosophical Transactions of the Royal Society B: Biological Sciences, 360(1462): 1847–1857.

Index

For Product Safety Concerns and Information please contact our EU
representative GPSR@taylorandfrancis.com
Taylor & Francis Verlag GmbH, Kaufingerstraße 24, 80331 München, Germany

www.ingramcontent.com/pod-product-compliance
Lightning Source LLC
Chambersburg PA
CBHW070714220326
41598CB00024BA/3149

9 7 8 1 0 3 2 2 1 0 9 7 1